SUPPLEMENT II to

JAPANESE

PHARMACEUTICAL

EXCIPIENTS

2018

JPE2018

YAKUJI NIPPO, LTD.

Supplement II to Japanese Pharmaceutical Excipients 2018 (Supplement II to JPE 2018)
英文版　医薬品添加物規格 2018　追補 II
　　ISBN978-4-8408-1609-0 C3047

Printed in Japan

PSEHB Notification No. 0307-1

March 7, 2022

To: Prefectural Governors

Director-General of Pharmaceutical Safety and Environmental Health Bureau,

Ministry of Health, Labour and Welfare

Partial Revision of "Japanese Pharmaceutical Excipients 2018"

The standards for pharmaceutical excipients are provided in Attachment entitled "Japanese Pharmaceutical Excipients 2018" (hereinafter referred to as "JPE 2018") of the notification "On Japanese Pharmaceutical Excipients 2018" (PSEHB Notification No. 0329-1 issued by the Director-General of Pharmaceutical Safety and Environmental Health Bureau, the Ministry of Health, Labour and Welfare dated March 29, 2018).

We hereby notify a partial revision of JPE 2018 as attached.

We ask you to understand an outline of the partial revision of JPE 2018 shown below together with the attachment and inform those of the relevant parties and organizations.

[Notice]

No.1   Outline of the partial revision of JPE 2018

　1   In accordance with the establishment of the Japanese Pharmacopoeia 18th edition, the general notices of JPE 2018 were revised.

　2   In General Tests, Processes and Apparatus, the following revisions were made:

　　(1)   The following items were revised.

　　　1)   Reagents, Test Solutions

　　　2)   Standard Solutions

　3   In the monographs of JPE 2018, the following revisions were made:

　　(1)   The specifications, etc. of the following items were revised.

1) Carboxyvinyl Polymer
2) Diethyl Phthalate
3) Glyceryl Monomyristate
4) Glyceryl Monooleate
5) Glyceryl Monostearate, Self-emulsifying Type
6) Hard Fat
7) Hydrophilic Hydrocarbon Gel
8) Maleated Rosin Glycerin Ester
9) D-Mannitol and Corn Starch Granules
10) Medium Chain Fatty Acid Triglyceride
11) Methacrylic Acid Copolymer LD
12) 2,2',2''-Nitrilotriethanol
13) Peru Balsam
14) Polyoxyethylene Castor Oil
15) Polyoxyethylene Glyceryl Monococoate (7E.O.)
16) Polyoxyethylene Glyceryl Triisostearate
17) Polyoxyethylene Hydrogenated Castor Oil 5
18) Polyoxyethylene Hydrogenated Castor Oil 10
19) Polyoxyethylene Hydrogenated Castor Oil 20
20) Polyoxyethylene Hydrogenated Castor Oil 40
21) Polyoxyethylene Hydrogenated Castor Oil 50
22) Polyoxyethylene Hydrogenated Castor Oil 60
23) Polyoxyethylene Hydrogenated Castor Oil 100
24) Polyoxyl 35 Castor Oil
25) Polyvinyl Chloride
26) Sucralose
27) α-Thioglycerol
28) Triacetine
29) Wheat Germ Oil

No.2　Schedule of Enforcement

This notification shall be applied on March 7, 2022. However, the standards then in force may remain applicable before and on September 30, 2023.

CONTENTS

CONTENTS

SUPPLEMENT II TO JAPANESE PHARMACEUTICAL EXCIPIENTS 2018

GENERAL NOTICES

1. These standards have been established for determination of the essence, method of preparation, description, quality and storage of a pharmaceutical excipient specified in JPE Monographs, and whether this pharmaceutical excipient is appropriate or not is tested as specified in General Notices; General Tests, Processes and Apparatus; and JPE monographs. However, the headings of "Description" in JPE Monographs are given for information, and should not be taken as indicating standards for conformity.

2. Unless otherwise specified in General Notices; General Tests, Processes and Apparatus; and JPE Monographs, the provisions of Paragraph 6, Paragraph 8 to Paragraph 11, and Paragraph 14 to Paragraph 48 inclusive, General Notices; General Tests, Processes and Apparatus of the Japanese Pharmacopoeia shall apply *mutatis mutandis* to these standards.

3. The title names and the commonly used names of drugs adopted in JPE Monographs should be used as official names. In JPE Monographs, English names are given for information.

4. The name of a drug marked with '   ' indicates a pharmaceutical excipient listed in JPE Monographs.

5. The name of a drug followed by (JP) indicates a drug listed in Japanese Pharmacopoeia.

6. The name of a drug marked with <   > in the section of Reference Standards, Reagents, Test Solutions, Standard Solutions for Volumetric Analysis and Standard Solutions indicates a pharmaceutical excipient specified in JPE Monographs which uses the relevant Reference Standard, Reagent, Test Solution, Standard Solution for Volumetric Analysis or Standard Solution.

7. The item name asterisked (*) in the section of Reference Standards, Reagents, Test Solutions, Standard Solutions for Volumetric Analysis and Standard Solutions indicates those of the same name in JP but different in the method of preparation.

GENERAL TESTS, PROCESSES AND APPARATUS

(3)　Reagents, Test Solutions

Change the following as follows:

Inositol for assay　It meets the requirements in description, identification, melting point, (1) Clarity and color of solution, (2) Chloride, (3) Sulfate, (4) Heavy metals, (5) Iron, (6) Calcium, (7) Arsenic, (8) Saccharide in Purity, Loss on drying and Residue on ignition of "Inositol", and the following tests.

Purity　Related substances－Dissolve 0.2 g of inositol for assay in 20 mL of water, and use this solution as the sample solution. Pipet 1 mL of this solution, add water to make exactly 100 mL, and use this solution as the standard solution. Perform the test with 10 μL each of the sample solution and standard solution as directed under Liquid Chromatography according to the following conditions. Determine each peak area of both solutions by the automatic integration method: the total area of the peaks other than inositol from the sample solution is not larger than the peak area of inositol from the standard solution.

Operating conditions －

　Proceed as directed in the Assay except the time span of measurement.

　Time span of measurement: About 3 times as long as the retention time of inositol, beginning after the solvent peak.

System suitability －

　Test for required detectability: Pipet 1mL of the standard solution, and add water to make exactly 10 mL. Confirm that the peak area of inositol obtained from 10 μL of this solution is equivalent to 7 to 13% of that from the standard solution.

　System performance: When the procedure is run with 10 μm of a mixture of 5 mL each of a solution of 1-propanol (1 in 3200) and the standard solution under the above operating conditions, inositol and 1-propanol are eluted in this order with the resolution between these peaks being not less than 2.0.

System repeatability: When the test is repeated 6 times with 10 μL of the standard solution under the above operating conditions, the relative standard deviation of the peak area of inositol is not more than 1.0%.

<Inositol>

(5)   Standard Solutions

Change the following as follows:

Standard Manganese Solution   Weigh exactly 3.60 g of manganese chloride (K8160, MnCl$_2$.4H$_2$O), dissolve in 50 mL of water and 10 mL of hydrochloric acid, and add water to make exactly 1000 mL. Pipet 10 mL of this solution, and dilute with water to make exactly 1000 mL: 1 mL of this solution contains 0.01 mg of manganese (Mn).

<Iron (III) Chloride Hydrate>

MONOGRAPHS FOR
SUPPLEMENT II TO JPE 2018

Change the following as follows:

101243

Carboxyvinyl Polymer

Carboxypolymethylene

カルボキシビニルポリマー

Carboxyvinyl Polymer is an acrylic acid polymer.

When dried, it contains not less than 58.0% and not more than 63.0% of carboxyl group (COOH: 45.02).

Description   Carboxyvinyl Polymer occurs as a white powder. It is odorless, or has a faint, characteristic odor, and has an acid taste.

It is practically insoluble in diethyl ether.

On the dispersion of Carboxyvinyl Polymer in water, in ethanol (95) and in *N,N*-dimethylformamide: it swells, and produces a clear or white-turbid, viscous liquid.

Identification

(1)   Disperse 0.5 g of Carboxyvinyl Polymer in 100 mL of water, add 2 drops of bromothymol blue TS, and add sodium hydroxide TS with stirring until a blue color develops: a strongly viscous liquid or gel is produced.

(2)   To about 10 mL of the liquid or gel obtained in (1) add 1 mL of calcium chloride TS, and stir: a white precipitate is formed immediately.

(3)   To about 10 mL of the liquid or gel obtained in (1) add 1 mL of magnesium sulfate TS, and stir: a white precipitate is formed immediately.

(4)   Determine the infrared absorption spectrum of Carboxyvinyl Polymer, previously dried, as directed in the potassium bromide disk method under Infrared Spectrophotometry: it exhibits absorption at the wave numbers of about 2960 cm^{-1}, 1720 cm^{-1}, 1455 cm^{-1}, 1415 cm^{-1}, 1250 cm^{-1}, 1175 cm^{-1} and 800 cm^{-1}.

Viscosity

(1)   Apparatus－Use a Brookfield type rotational viscosimeter illustrated in the figure.

Brookfield type rotational viscosimeter

Figures are in mm.

Table of viscosity standards

Viscosity of the sample solution	Rotor	Calculation multiplier
Less than 10,000 mPa·s	I (No. 4)	100
10,000 mPa·s or more	J (No. 6)	500

A: Synchronous motor   F: Pointer

B: Change gear and clutch   G: Dipping mark

C: Lever   H: Rotor

D: Scale plate   I: No. 4 rotor

E: Joint   J: No. 6 rotor

(2)　Procedure—Take 0.40 g of Carboxyvinyl Polymer, previously dried, transfer it to a 200-mL beaker containing 200 mL of water, and disperse, preventing from bubbling. While stirring, adjust the pH of this solution with sodium hydroxide TS to 7.0 to 7.5, allow to stand for more than 10 hours to remove bubbles, and use this solution as the sample solution. According to the table of viscosity standards, attach rotor I or J to joint E, dip the rotor in the sample solution to dipping mark G while preventing bubbles from adhering, and turn the rotor at 20 rpm. Keep the temperature of the sample solution at 20 ± 0.1°C. Push lever C after 30 seconds to fix pointer F, stop the turning of the rotor, read the pointer on scale plate D, and multiply by the calculation multiplier shown in the table of viscosity standards. Make reading with 3 sample solutions, and calculate the average: it is 1500 to 50,000 mPa·s.

pH   Disperse 0.20 g of Carboxyvinyl Polymer in 100 mL of freshly boiled and cooled water: the pH of this dispersion is between 2.5 and 4.0.

Purity

(1)   Heavy metals—To 2.0 g of Carboxyvinyl Polymer in a platinum, quartz or porcelain crucible add 20 mL of a solution of magnesium nitrate hexahydrate in ethanol (95) (1 in 20), fire the ethanol to burn, and heat gradually to carbonize. After cooling, add 1 mL of sulfuric acid, heat carefully, and then heat strongly at 500°C to 600°C to incinerate. If a carbonized substance still remains with this method, moisten it with a small quantity of sulfuric acid, and heat strongly to incinerate. After cooling, dissolve the residue in 3 mL of hydrochloric acid, evaporate on a water bath to dryness, and dissolve the residue in 10 mL of water by warming. To this solution add 1 drop of phenolphthalein TS, then add ammonia TS dropwise until a pale red color develops, add 2 mL of dilute acetic acid, filter if necessary, and wash the filter with 10 mL of water. Transfer the filtrate and washing to a Nessler tube, and add water to make 50 mL. Perform the test using this solution as the test solution. Prepare the control solution as follows: proceed with 20 mL of a solution of magnesium nitrate hexahydrate in ethanol (95) (1 in 20) in the same manner as the preparation of the test solution, and add 2.0 mL of Standard Lead Solution and water to make 50 mL (not more than 10 ppm).

(2)   Arsenic—To 2.5 g of Carboxyvinyl Polymer add gradually 20 mL of nitric acid, and heat gently until the solution is fluidized. After cooling, add 5 mL of sulfuric acid, and heat until brown fumes are no longer evolved. Add occasionally a 2- to 3- mL portion of nitric acid, and heat until the solution becomes colorless to pale yellow. After cooling, add 15 mL of a saturated solution of ammonium oxalate monohydrate, and heat until white fumes are evolved. After cooling, add water to make 25 mL. Perform the test with 10 mL of this solution as the test solution (not more than 2 ppm).

(3)   Free acrylic acid—Weigh accurately about 1.0 g of Carboxyvinyl Polymer in an iodine bottle, add 100 mL of water, and allow to stand for about 24 hours to disperse with occasional shaking. To this dispersion add exactly 10 mL of 0.05 mol/L bromine VS, then add 20 mL of diluted hydrochloric acid (1 in 2), immediately stopper the vessel tightly, shake well, and allow to stand in a dark place for 20 minutes. To this solution add carefully 20 mL of potassium iodide TS, immediately stopper the vessel tightly, shake well, and titrate the liberated iodine with 0.1 mol/L sodium thiosulfate VS (indicator: 1 mL of starch TS). Perform a blank determination in the same manner. The amount of free acrylic acid is not more than 1.0%.

$$\text{Amount (\%) of free acrylic acid (C}_3\text{H}_4\text{O}_2) = \frac{(a-b) \times 0.3603}{\text{amount (g) of sample}}$$

where

a: Amount (mL) of 0.1 mol/L sodium thiosulfate VS consumed in the blank determination

b: Amount (mL) of 0.1 mol/L sodium thiosulfate VS consumed in the test of the sample

Loss on drying   Not more than 7.0% (2 g, 105°C, 3 hours).

Residue on ignition   Not more than 2.5% (1 g).

Assay   Weigh accurately about 0.1 g of Carboxyvinyl Polymer, previously dried, disperse in 100 mL of diluted *N,N*-dimethylformamide (3 in 10), and titrate with 0.1 mol/L potassium hydroxide-ethanol VS (potentiometric titration). Perform a blank determination in the same manner, and make any necessary correction.

Each mL of 0.1 mol/L potassium hydroxide-ethanol VS = 4.502 mg of COOH

Containers and storage   Containers—Well-closed containers.

Administration route   Oral administration, general external preparation, sublingual application, rectum vagina urethra application, ophthalmic preparation, dental external use and troche use, otorhinology preparation.

[Note: This item has been revised in the Japanese edition, but the revision does not require any change to the English text stated in the English edition.]

Change the following as follows:

101815

Diethyl Phthalate

フタル酸ジエチル

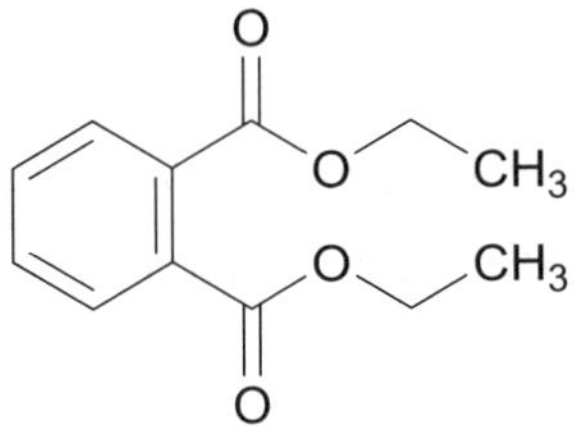

$C_{12}H_{14}O_4$: 222.24

Diethyl Phthalate contains not less than 99.0% of diethyl phthalate ($C_{12}H_{14}O_4$), calculated on the anhydrous basis.

Description   Diethyl Phthalate is a clear, colorless liquid. It is odorless, or has a faint, characteristic odor.

It is miscible with ethanol (95) and with diethyl ether, and very slightly soluble in water.

Identification   Determine the infrared absorption spectrum of Diethyl Phthalate as directed in the liquid film method under Infrared Spectrophotometry: it exhibits absorption at the wave numbers of about 1729 cm^{-1}, 1600 cm^{-1}, 1285 cm^{-1}, 1124 cm^{-1} and 745 cm^{-1}.

Refractive index n_D^{20}: 1.499−1.504

Specific gravity d_{20}^{20}: 1.118−1.125

Acid value   Not more than 0.1.

Purity

(1)   Heavy metals−Proceed with 1.0 g of Diethyl Phthalate according to Method 2, and perform the test. Prepare the control solution with 2.0 mL of Standard Lead Solution (not more than 20 ppm).

(2)   Arsenic−Prepare the test solution with 1.0 g of Diethyl Phthalate according to Method 3, and perform the test (not more than 2 ppm).

Water   Not more than 0.5 g/dL (1 mL, coulometric titration).

Residue on ignition   Not more than 0.10% (5 g).

Assay Weigh accurately about 1 g of Diethyl Phthalate, add exactly 50 mL of 0.5 mol/L potassium hydroxide-ethanol VS, heat under a reflux condenser on a water bath for 2 hours, cool, and titrate with 0.5 mol/L hydrochloric acid VS (indicator: 1 mL of phenolphthalein TS). Perform a blank determination in the same manner.

Each mL of 0.5 mol/L potassium hydroxide-ethanol VS = 55.56 mg of $C_{12}H_{14}O_4$

Containers and storage Containers — Tight containers.
Administration route Oral administration.

[Note: This item has been revised in the Japanese edition, but the revision does not require any change to the English text stated in the English edition.]

Change the following as follows:

102541

Glyceryl Monomyristate

モノミリスチン酸グリセリン

Glyceryl Monomyristate consists mainly of monomyristate ester of glycerin.

Description   Glyceryl Monomyristate occurs as white to pale yellow, waxy masses or flake.

It is very slightly soluble in ethanol (99.5), and practically insoluble in water.

Identification

(1)   To 0.2 g of Glyceryl Monomyristate add 10 mL of water, warm, and mix by thorough shaking. After cooling, add 5 drops of bromine TS: the color of the test solution does not disappear.

(2)   Determine the infrared absorption spectrum of Glyceryl Monomyristate as directed in the liquid film method under Infrared Spectrophotometry: it exhibits absorption at the wave numbers of about 3410 cm^{-1}, 2920 cm^{-1}, 2850 cm^{-1}, 1738 cm^{-1}, 1467 cm^{-1}, 1178 cm^{-1} and 721 cm^{-1}.

Melting point   44－48°C (Method 2).

Acid value   10－20

Saponification value   190－210

Purity   Heavy metals－Proceed with 1.0 g of Glyceryl Monomyristate according to Method 2, and perform the test. Prepare the control solution with 2.0 mL of Standard Lead Solution (not more than 20 ppm).

Water   Not more than 3.0% (1 g, direct titration).

Residue on ignition   Not more than 0.5% (1 g).

Containers and storage   Containers－Tight containers.

Administration route   Rectum vagina urethra application.

Change the following as follows:

122110

Glyceryl Monooleate

モノオレイン酸グリセリン

Glyceryl Monooleate consists chiefly of glyceryl monooleate, and also contains glyceryl dioleate, glyceryl trioleate and unreacted glycerin.

Description Glyceryl Monooleate occurs as pale yellow to yellow liquid or petrolatum-like substance. It has a faint, characteristic odor.

It is freely soluble in methanol, in ethanol (95) and in diethyl ether, and practically insoluble in water.

Identification Dissolve 0.1 g of Glyceryl Monooleate in 2 mL of ethanol (95) by warming, heat with 5 mL of dilute sulfuric acid on a water bath for 30 minutes, and cool: a light yellow to brown oily substance is separated. To this substance add 3 mL of diethyl ether, and shake: it dissolves.

Acid Value Not more than 5.0.

Saponification value 150－175

Iodine value 65－80

Purity Heavy metals－Proceed with 1.0 g of Glyceryl Monooleate according to Method 2, and perform the test. Prepare the control solution with 2.0 mL of Standard Lead Solution (not more than 20 ppm).

Water Not more than 0.5% (1 g, direct titration).

Residue on ignition Not more than 0.5% (1 g).

Containers and storage Containers－Tight containers.

Administration route General external preparation.

Change the following as follows:

102543

Glyceryl Monostearate, Self-emulsifying Type

自己乳化型モノステアリン酸グリセリン

Glyceryl Monostearate, Self-emulsifying Type is prepared as follows: to mainly glyceryl monostearate add soap or hydrophilic non-ionic surfactant to increase hydrophilic nature.

Description   Glyceryl Monostearate, Self-emulsifying Type occurs as white to pale yellow masses or thin flake. It has a faint, characteristic odor.

It is freely soluble in or slightly soluble in chloroform, very slightly soluble in or practically insoluble in ethanol (95), and practically insoluble in water.

Identification

(1)   To 5 g of Glyceryl Monostearate, Self-emulsifying Type add 100 mL of water, heat until the sample is liquid, shake vigorously, and allow to stand: an oily layer does not separate.

(2)   To 0.1 g of Glyceryl Monostearate, Self-emulsifying Type add 2 mL of ethanol (95), dissolve by warming, add 5 mL of dilute sulfuric acid, heat on a water bath for 30 minutes, and cool: a yellow-white solid is formed. Separate this solid, and shake with 3 mL of diethyl ether: it dissolves.

Melting point   50－65°C (Method 2).

Acid value   Not more than 20.

Saponification value   90－160

Purity

(1)   Glycerin－Weigh accurately about 1 g of Glyceryl Monostearate, Self-emulsifying Type, add 20 mL of chloroform, and dissolve by warming. After cooling, transfer to a separator, and extract with three 25-mL portions of a solution of acetic acid (100) (2 in 25). Transfer the extract to an iodine bottle. To this extract add exactly 20 mL of periodic acid TS, shake, allow to stand for 15 minutes, add 10 mL of a solution of potassium iodide (1 in 4), and immediately titrate with 0.2 mol/L sodium thiosulfate VS: it is not more than 10.0%. Perform a blank determination in the same manner, and make any necessary correction (indicator: 3 mL of starch TS).

Each mL of 0.2 mol/L sodium thiosulfate VS = 4.605 mg of $C_3H_8O_3$

(2)   Heavy metals—Proceed with 1.0 g of Glyceryl Monostearate, Self-emulsifying Type according to Method 2, and perform the test. Prepare the control solution with 2.0 mL of Standard Lead Solution (not more than 20 ppm).

Water   Not more than 5.0% (1 g, direct titration).

Residue on ignition   Not more than 4.0% (1 g).

Containers and storage   Containers—Tight containers.
    Storage—Light-resistant.

Administration route   General external preparation.

Change the following as follows:

108544

Hard Fat

ハードファット

Hard Fat is mainly composed of a triglyceride of saturated fatty acid [$CH_3(CH_2)_nCOOH$, where *n* is 6 to 16].

Description   Hard Fat occurs as a white to pale yellow, waxy solid. It is odorless, or has a faint, characteristic odor, and is tasteless.

Melt Hard Fat by warming: it becomes a colorless to light yellow liquid.

It is miscible with diethyl ether.

It is slightly soluble in ethanol (95), and practically insoluble in water.

Identification   To 0.1 g of Hard Fat add 2 mL of ethanol (95), dissolve by warming, add 5 mL of dilute sulfuric acid, heat in a water bath for 30 minutes, and cool: a white to yellow-white solid separates out. Collect this solid, and shake with 3 mL of diethyl ether: it dissolves.

Melting point $30-45°C$

Acid value   Not more than 2.0.

Saponification value $210-255$

Hydroxyl value   Not more than 70.

Unsaponifiable matter   Not more than 3.0%.

Iodine value   Not more than 3.0. Use 10 mL of a mixture of acetic acid (100) and cyclohexane (1:1) instead of cyclohexane as solvent.

Purity

(1)   Water and coloration－Melt 5.0 g of Hard Fat by heating on a water bath: the liquid obtained is clear, and does not separate water. View this liquid in a 10-mm layer: it is colorless to pale yellow.

(2)   Alkalinity－To 2.0 g of Hard Fat add 10 mL of water, melt by warming on a water bath, and shake vigorously. After cooling, to the water layer separated add 1 drop of phenolphthalein TS: the solution is colorless.

(3)   Heavy metals－Proceed with 2.0 g of Hard Fat according to Method 2, and perform the test. Prepare the control solution with 2.0 mL of Standard Lead Solution (not more than 10 ppm).

(4) Arsenic — Prepare the test solution with 1.0 g of Hard Fat according to Method 3, and perform the test (not more than 2 ppm).

Residue on ignition Not more than 0.10% (1 g).

Containers and storage Containers — Well-closed containers.

Administration route General external preparation, percutaneous, rectum vagina urethra application.

Change the following as follows:

120267

Hydrophilic Hydrocarbon Gel

親水ゲル化炭化水素

Hydrophilic Hydrocarbon Gel is obtained by adding glycerol esters of fatty acids to 'Hydrocarbon Gel' to give a hydrophile.

Description   Hydrophilic Hydrocarbon Gel occurs as a translucent, white to whitish, petrolatum-like substance. It is odorless, or has a faint, characteristic odor.

It is practically insoluble in water, in ethanol (95) and in diethyl ether.

Identification

(1)   Place Hydrophilic Hydrocarbon Gel on a porcelain dish, and fire by strong heating: it burns with a bright flame, and the odor of paraffin vapor is perceptible.

(2)   To 10 g of Hydrophilic Hydrocarbon Gel add 30 mL of diethyl ether, shake, and filter. Wash the residue with three 30-mL portions of diethyl ether, air-dry, and dissolve about 0.2 g of the residue in 3 mL of xylene by warming on a water bath. Drop this solution on a clean glass plate, evaporate the xylene by warming on a water bath to make film, and determine the infrared absorption spectrum as directed in the film method under Infrared Spectrophotometry: it exhibits absorption at the wave numbers of about 2920 cm^{-1}, 2850 cm^{-1}, 1464 cm^{-1}, 1377 cm^{-1} and 719 cm^{-1}.

(3)   To 10 g of Hydrophilic Hydrocarbon Gel add 50 mL of ethanol (95), and warm under a reflux condenser on a water bath for 30 minutes with shaking. Separate the ethanol layer while warming, evaporate ethanol on a water bath, add 2 mL of ethanol (95) to the residue so obtained, dissolve it by warming, add 5 mL of dilute sulfuric acid, heat in a water bath for 30 minutes, and cool: an oil drop or a white to yellow-white solid separates out.

Specific gravity d_{20}^{20}: $0.870-0.900$. (Proceed as directed in the Specific gravity under Fats and Fatty Oils Test).

Acid value   Not more than 0.3.

Purity

(1)   Acidity or alkalinity－To 10.0 g of Hydrophilic Hydrocarbon Gel add 10 mL of hot water

and 1 drop of phenolphthalein TS, heat in a water bath for 5 minutes, and shake vigorously: no red color develops. To this solution add 0.20 mL of 0.02 mol/L sodium hydroxide VS, and shake: a red color develops.

(2)   Heavy metals — Proceed with 2.0 g of Hydrophilic Hydrocarbon Gel according to Method 2, and perform the test. Prepare the control solution with 2.0 mL of Standard Lead Solution (not more than 10 ppm).

(3)   Polyoxyethylene — Boil 10 g of Hydrophilic Hydrocarbon Gel with 50 mL of water, cool, and filter. Add 10 mL of ammonium thiocyanate-cobalt (II) nitrate TS to the filtrate, shake well, then shake with 10 mL of chloroform, and allow to stand: the chloroform layer does not develop a blue color.

(4)   Free liquid paraffin — Pack evenly and possibly free of air Hydrophilic Hydrocarbon Gel in a tared cylindrical vessel (45 mm in inside diameter and 40 mm in height) using a spatula, make the surface flat, insert a triangle ruler with the 90° vertex near the central point of the vessel, rotate the triangle ruler slowly to cut out an inverted cone with the upper part of the vessel as its base and the 90° angle as the vertex, and weigh it accurately. Cover the vessel, allow to stand at 45°C for 15 hours, collect, while hot, the liquid paraffin gathered in the vertex of the hollow in the form of inverted cone, and weigh it accurately: it is not more than 0.2%.

Residue on ignition   Not more than 0.5% (1 g).

Containers and storage   Containers — Tight containers.

Administration route   General external preparation.

Change the following as follows:

120064

Maleated Rosin Glycerin Ester

マレイン化ロジングリセリンエステル

Maleated Rosin Glycerin Ester is obtained from the following process: to rosin 12 to 14% of Glycerin (JP) and 7 to 9% of maleic anhydride is added to react for esterification, from which unreacted glycerin and maleic anhydride are removed under reduced pressure, and made it to flake after cooling.

Description   Maleated Rosin Glycerin Ester occurs as light yellow, transparent flakes. It is odorless, or has a faint, characteristic odor.

It is freely soluble in acetone and in diethyl ether, slightly soluble in ethanol (95) and in acetic anhydride, and practically insoluble in water.

Identification

(1)   To 0.1 g of powdered Maleated Rosin Glycerin Ester add 10 mL of acetic anhydride, dissolve it on a water bath by heating, cool, and add 1 drop of sulfuric acid: a purple-red color develops immediately.

(2)   To 1 g of powdered Maleated Rosin Glycerin Ester add 5 mL of sodium hydroxide TS and 5 mL of water, and shake vigorously: the solution shows a light yellow turbidity, and persistent foams are produced.

(3)   Determine the infrared absorption spectrum of Maleated Rosin Glycerin Ester as directed in the potassium bromide disk method under Infrared Spectrophotometry: it exhibits absorption at the wave numbers of about 1850 cm^{-1}, 1780 cm^{-1}, 1730 cm^{-1}, 1225 cm^{-1} and 1130 cm^{-1}.

Softening point   120－130°C

(1)   Apparatus－Use the apparatuses illustrated in in Figs. 1 to 5.

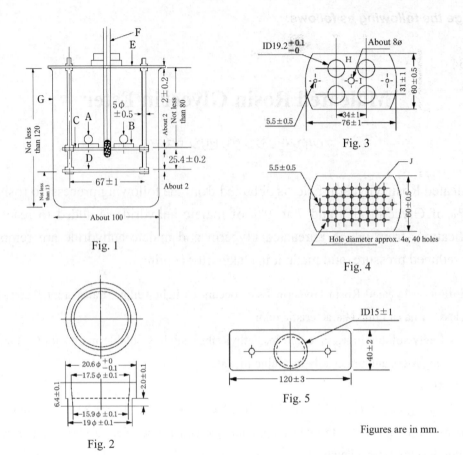

Fig. 1

Fig. 2

Fig. 3

Fig. 4

Fig. 5

Figures are in mm.

A: Steel ball (diameter: 9.5 mm, weight: 3.5 g)

B: Ring (brass, illustrated in Fig. 2)

C: Ring-supporting plate (metal, as roughly illustrated in Fig. 3)

D: Bottom plate (illustrated in Fig. 4, having 40 convection holes J)

E: Setting plate (illustrated in Fig. 5)

F: Thermometer No. 1 (place the center of the mercury bulb as high as the lower plane of the ring-supporting plate C)

G: Glass vessel

H: Supporting hole for the ring

I: Insert hole for the mercury bulb of thermometer

J: Convection hole (diameter: about 4 mm)

(2) Procedure－Melt the sample at the temperature as low as possible, place the ring B on the flat metal plate, fill carefully the melted sample in B so that foam may not enter, allow to stand for 40 minutes at room temperature, and cut off the swelling portion from the plane containing upper surface of B with a slightly heated knife. Pour silicone oil into glass vessel G up to more than 90-mm depth, and keep it at the temperature about 60°C below the expected softening point. Put the steel ball A on the center of the sample surface in B, and fix B in the supporting holes H. Then set the distance between the upper surface of B and the silicone oil at 50 ± 2 mm, allow to stand for 15 to 20 minutes, and start to heat. Keep heating so as to raise the temperature at the rate of 5 ± 0.5°C per minute. Measure the temperature as softening point, when the sample is gradually softened, followed down from B, and reaches the bottom plate D. The measurement is performed more than twice using 4 pieces of B for each time, and the average value is calculated.

Acid value   19－24

Purity   Heavy metals － Proceed with 1.0 g of powdered Maleated Rosin Glycerin Ester according to Method 2, and perform the test. Prepare the control solution with 2.0 mL of Standard Lead Solution (not more than 20 ppm).

Residue on ignition   Not more than 0.10% (1 g).

Containers and storage   Containers－Tight containers.

Administration route   General external preparation.

Change the following as follows:

890032

D-Mannitol and Corn Starch Granules

D－マンニトール・トウモロコシデンプン造粒物

D-Mannitol and Corn Starch Granules is the granules of D-Mannitol (JP) and Corn Starch (JP), which is mixed and granulated.

It contains not less than 78.0% and not more than 82.0% of D-mannitol ($C_6H_{14}O_6$: 182.17) and not less than 15.0% and not more than 19.0% of corn starch.

Description D-Mannitol and Corn Starch Granules occurs as a white, granulated powder.

Identification

  (1) Determine the infrared absorption spectrum of D-Mannitol and Corn Starch Granules as directed in the potassium bromide disk method under Infrared Spectrophotometry, and compare the spectrum with the Reference Spectrum of D-Mannitol in the Japanese Pharmacopoeia or the spectrum of D-Mannitol RS: both spectra exhibit similar intensities of absorption at the same wave numbers. If any difference appears between the spectra, put 25 mg each of D-Mannitol and Corn Starch Granules and D-Mannitol RS in glass vessels, dissolve the components of D-mannitol in 0.25 mL of water without heating, dry them in a 600－700 W microwave oven for 20 minutes or in a drying chamber at 100°C for 1 hour, then further dry by gradual reducing pressure, and perform the same test as above with so obtained non-sticky white to pale yellow powders: both spectra exhibit similar intensities of absorption at the same wave numbers.

  (2) Examined under a microscope, using mixture of water and glycerin (1:1), D-Mannitol and Corn Starch Granules appears as either angular polyhedral granules of irregular sizes with diameters of 2－23 μm or as rounded or spheroidal granules of irregular sizes with diameters of 25－35 μm. The central hilum consists of a distinct cavity or two- to five-rayed cleft, and there are no concentric striations. Between orthogonally oriented polarizing plates or prisms, the starch granules show a distinct black cross intersecting at the hilum.

  (3) To 1 g of D-Mannitol and Corn Starch Granules add 50 mL of water, boil for 1 minute, and allow to cool: a thin, cloudy mucilage is formed. To 1 mL of the mucilage add 0.05 mL of diluted iodine TS (1 in 10): an orange-red to deep blue color is formed and the color disappears by heating.

Purity Sulfur dioxide (SO_2)－Suspend 20 g of D-Mannitol and Corn Starch Granules in 200 mL of water, and stir. Allow to stand for 2 to 3 minutes, stir again, and filter. To 100 mL of the filtrate add 4 to 5 mL of starch TS, and titrate with 0.005 mol/L iodine VS. Perform a blank determination in the same manner, and make any necessary correction. Calculate the amount of sulfur dioxide: it is not more than 10 ppm.

$$\text{Amount (ppm) of sulfur dioxide} = \frac{V}{M} \times 640$$

M: Amount (g) of sample

V: Volume (mL) of 0.005 mol/L iodine VS consumed

Each mL of 0.005 mol/L iodine VS consumed = 0.32 mg of SO_2

Loss on drying Not more than 3.0% (5 g, 130°C, 90 minutes).

Residue on ignition Place about 1 g of D-Mannitol and Corn Starch Granules in a tared crucible, and weigh accurately. Moisten the sample with 2 mL of diluted sulfuric acid (11 in 200), heat gradually at the temperature as low as possible, and carbonize the sample completely. Heat strongly at 600 ± 25°C, and incinerate the residue. Allow to cool, add several drops of a solution of ammonium carbonate (79 in 500), heat gradually until white fumes are no longer evolved, and incinerate again. Cool the crucible in a desiccator, weigh accurately and calculate the percentage of residue: it is not more than 0.2%.

Particle size Perform the test employing No. 50 (300 μm) and 100 μm sieves with the inside diameter of 200 mm. Weigh accurately 50 g of sample to be tested, and place on the top (coarse) sieve of the nest of sieves described above and the collecting pan and place the lid. Shake the sieves in a horizontal direction for 3 minutes, and tap slightly at intervals. Weigh the amount remaining on each sieve and in the receiving pan: not less than 80% of the total amount remains in the 100 μm sieve, and not more than 20% remains in the No. 50 (300 μm) sieve.

Assay

(1) D-Mannitol－Weigh accurately about 0.8 g of D-Mannitol and Corn Starch Granules, add 25 mL of water, and boil for 3 minutes. To this solution add water to make 50 mL. After cooling, add water to make exactly 100 mL, filter through a membrane filter with a pore size not exceeding 0.45 μm, and use this solution as the sample solution. Separately, weigh accurately 1 g of D-Mannitol RS as described in the Reference Standards in JP (separately determine the loss on drying in the same conditions as D-Mannitol (JP)), dissolve in water

to make exactly 50 mL, and use this solution as the standard stock solution. Pipet 1 mL, 5 mL and 10 mL of the standard stock solution, add water to make them exactly 20 mL, and use these solutions as the standard solution (1), (2) and (3). Perform the test with exactly 20 μL each of the sample solution, standard solution (1), (2) and (3) as directed under Liquid Chromatography according to the following conditions. Prepare the calibration curve by plotting the concentration of D-mannitol and the peak area from the standard solution of mannitol, determine the concentration, C (g/mL), of D-mannitol in the sample solution, and calculate the amount (%) of D-mannitol by the following equation.

$$\text{Amount (\%) of D-mannitol in sample} = \frac{C}{X} \times 10,000$$

X: Amount (g) of sample

Operating conditions —

Detector: A differential refractometer.

Column: A stainless steel column 7.8 mm in inside diameter and 30 cm in length, packed with strongly acidic ion-exchange resin (Ca type) for liquid chromatography composed with a sulfonated polystyrene cross-linked with divinylbenzene (9 μm in particle diameter).

Column temperature: 85°C

Mobile phase: Water

Flow rate: 0.5 mL per minute.

System suitability —

System performance: When the procedure is run with 20 μL of the standard solution (2) under the above operating conditions, the number of theoretical plates and the symmetry factor of the peak of D-mannitol are not less than 6000, and not more than 0.8 to 1.5, respectively.

System repeatability: When the test is repeated 6 times with 20 μL of the standard solution (2) under the above operating conditions, the relative standard deviation of the peak area of D-mannitol is not more than 1.0%.

(2) Corn Starch—Determine the total optical rotation and the optical rotation of the sample solution in diluted ethanol (99.5) (1 in 10), and calculate the amount of corn starch.

(i) Determination of total optical rotation: Weigh accurately about 2.5 g of D-Mannitol and Corn Starch Granules, add 50 mL of diluted hydrochloric acid (133 in 5000), and stir to make uniform suspension. For the first 3 minutes, stir vigorously at a constant rate, to avoid aggregation, while heating in a water bath, and then stir for an additional 12 minutes. Take the solution out of the water bath, and cool to 20°C in running water. Add 5 mL of Carrez TS I, stir for 1 minute, add 5 mL of Carrez TS II, and then stir again for 1 minute. To this suspension add water to make exactly 100 mL, filter, and determine the optical rotation in 100-mm cell at 20 ± 1°C as directed under Optical Rotation Determination.

(ii) Determination of optical rotation of the sample solution in diluted ethanol (99.5): Weigh accurately about 5 g of D-Mannitol and Corn Starch Granules, and add about 80 mL of diluted ethanol (99.5) (1 in 10). Warm the suspension under a reflux condenser at 50°C for 30 minutes, and, after 30 minutes, cool at room temperature while shaking. To this suspension add diluted ethanol (99.5) (1 in 10) to make exactly 100 mL, and filter. To 50 mL of the filtrate (equivalent to 2.5 g of sample) add 2.1 mL of diluted hydrochloric acid (663 in 1000), and mix well. Heat the solution under a reflux condenser for 15 minutes, and cool rapidly to 20°C. Add 5 mL of Carrez TS I, shake for 1 minute, add 5 mL of Carrez TS II, and then shake for 1 minute. To this solution add water to make exactly 100 mL, filter, and determine the optical rotation in 100-mm cell at 20 ± 1°C as directed under Optical Rotation Determination.

(iii) Calculation method:

$$\text{Content (\%) of starch in sample} = \frac{P \times \left(\frac{2.5}{M_1}\right) - P' \times \left(\frac{5}{M_2}\right)}{+184.6} \times 4000$$

M_1: Amount (g) of sample in (i)
M_2: Amount (g) of sample in (ii)
P: Total optical rotation (°) obtained in (i)
P': Optical rotation (°) obtained in (ii)
+184.6: Optical rotation (°) of corn starch

Containers and storage Containers—Well-closed containers.
Administration route Oral administration.

Change the following as follows:

109201

Medium Chain Fatty Acid Triglyceride

中鎖脂肪酸トリグリセリド

Medium Chain Fatty Acid Triglyceride is mainly composed of a triglyceride of saturated fatty acid ($CH_3(CH_2)_nCOOH$, where n is 4 to 10).

Description Medium Chain Fatty Acid Triglyceride is a clear, colorless to pale yellow liquid. It is odorless, or has a faint, characteristic odor and a mild taste.

It is miscible with ethanol (95), with diethyl ether, with cyclohexane and with petroleum ether, and not miscible with water.

Identification Mix 0.1 g of Medium Chain Fatty Acid Triglyceride with 2 mL of ethanol (95), add 5 mL of dilute sulfuric acid, heat in a water bath for 30 minutes, and cool: the odor of lower fatty acid is perceptible.

Acid value Not more than 0.5.

Saponification value 320－385

Hydroxyl value Not more than 10.

Unsaponifiable matter Not more than 1.0%.

Iodine value Not more than 1.0.

Purity

(1) Alkalinity－To 2.0 g of Medium Chain Fatty Acid Triglyceride add 10 mL of water, warm in a water bath, and shake vigorously. After cooling, to the separated water layer add 1 drop of phenolphthalein TS: the solution is colorless.

(2) Heavy metals－Proceed with 2.0 g of Medium Chain Fatty Acid Triglyceride according to Method 2, and perform the test. Prepare the control solution with 2.0 mL of Standard Lead Solution (not more than 10 ppm).

(3) Arsenic－Prepare the test solution with 1.0 g of Medium Chain Fatty Acid Triglyceride according to Method 3, and perform the test (not more than 2 ppm).

Water Not more than 0.20% (2 g, direct titration).

Residue on ignition Not more than 0.10% (1 g).

Containers and storage Containers — Tight containers.

Administration route Oral administration, general external preparation, sublingual application.

Change the following as follows:

108617

Methacrylic Acid Copolymer LD

メタクリル酸コポリマーLD

Methacrylic Acid Copolymer LD is an emulsion of a copolymer of methacrylic acid and ethyl acrylate obtained in a solution of Polysorbate 80 (JP) and Sodium Lauryl Sulfate (JP).

It contains not less than 11.5% and not more than 15.5% of the copolymer structural components of methacrylic acid ($C_4H_6O_2$: 86.09).

Description   Methacrylic Acid Copolymer LD is a white emulsion. It has a characteristic odor and a slightly acid taste.

It is freely soluble in ethanol (95) and in acetone, and practically insoluble in diethyl ether.

It disperses homogeneously in water.

It dissolves in dilute sodium hydroxide TS.

Identification

(1)   To 0.5 mL of Methacrylic Acid Copolymer LD add 5 mL of dilute sodium hydroxide TS, and shake: the solution becomes a clear, viscous liquid. To this solution add 1 mL of dilute hydrochloric acid: a white, resinous precipitate is formed.

(2)   Thinly coat the optical plate with Methacrylic Acid Copolymer LD, and determine the infrared absorption spectrum of a thin film obtained by evaporating the solvent as directed in the film method under Infrared Spectrophotometry: it exhibits absorption at the wave numbers of about 2980 cm^{-1}, 1735 cm^{-1}, 1705 cm^{-1}, 1475 cm^{-1}, 1450 cm^{-1}, 1385 cm^{-1} and 1180 cm^{-1}.

(3)   To 5 mL of Methacrylic Acid Copolymer LD add 3 mL of ammonium thiocyanate-cobalt (II) nitrate TS, shake well, add 10 mL of chloroform, shake, and allow to stand: a light blue color develops in the chloroform layer.

Viscosity $3-15$ mm^2/s (Method 1, 20°C).

pH $2.1-3.1$

Specific gravity d_{20}^{20}: $1.055-1.080$

Purity

(1)   Heavy metals─Proceed with 2.0 g of Methacrylic Acid Copolymer LD according to Method 2, and perform the test. Prepare the control solution with 2.0 mL of Standard Lead Solution (not more than 10 ppm).

(2)   Arsenic ─ Prepare the test solution with 2.0 g of Methacrylic Acid Copolymer LD according to Method 3, and perform the test (not more than 1 ppm).

(3)   Methacrylic acid and ethyl acrylate─Weigh accurately about 10 g of Methacrylic Acid Copolymer LD, dissolve in methanol for liquid chromatography to make exactly 50 mL. Pipet 10 mL of this solution, put it into a container containing exactly 5 mL of a solution of sodium perchlorate monohydrate (7 in 200) with stirring, centrifuge, and use the supernatant liquid as the sample solution. Separately, weigh accurately about 10 mg each of methacrylic acid and ethyl acrylate, dissolve in 5 mL of 1-butanol, and add methanol for liquid chromatography to make exactly 50 mL. Pipet 5 mL of this solution, and add methanol for liquid chromatography to make exactly 50 mL. Pipet 5 mL of this solution, add methanol for liquid chromatography to make exactly 50 mL, and use this solution as the standard stock solution. Pipet 10 mL of the standard stock solution, add exactly 5 mL of a solution of sodium perchlorate monohydrate (7 in 200), and use this solution as the standard solution. Perform the test with exactly 20 µL each of the sample solution and standard solution as directed under Liquid Chromatography according to the following conditions, the peak area, A_{T1} and A_{T2}, of methacrylic acid and ethyl acrylate from the sample solution and the peak area, A_{S1} and A_{S2}, of methacrylic acid and ethyl acrylate from the standard solution, and calculate their amounts: the amount of methacrylic acid and ethyl acrylate is not more than 50 ppm, respectively.

$$\text{Amount (ppm) of methacrylic acid} = 10 \times \frac{M_{S1}}{M_T} \times \frac{A_{T1}}{A_{S1}}$$

$$\text{Amount (ppm) of ethyl acrylate} = 10 \times \frac{M_{S2}}{M_T} \times \frac{A_{T2}}{A_{S2}}$$

M_{S1}: Amount (mg) of methacrylic acid

M_{S2}: Amount (mg) of ethyl acrylate

M_T: Amount (g) of sample

Operating conditions ─

Detector: An ultraviolet absorption photometer (wavelength: 202 nm).

Column: A stainless steel column about 4.6 mm in inside diameter and about 12.5 cm in length, packed with octadecylsilanized silica gel for liquid chromatography (7 μm in particle diameter).

Column temperature: A constant temperature of about 20°C.

Mobile phase: A mixture of a solution of phosphoric acid (pH 2) and methanol for liquid chromatography (4:1).

Flow rate: Adjust so that the retention time of ethyl acrylate is about 7 minutes.

System suitability—

Test for required detectability: Pipet 2 mL of the standard stock solution, add methanol for liquid chromatography to make exactly 10 mL, and add exactly 5 mL of a solution of sodium perchlorate monohydrate (7 in 200). Confirm that the peak area of methacrylic acid and ethyl acrylate obtained from 20 μL of this solution is equivalent to 18 to 22% of that obtained from the standard solution.

System performance: When the procedure is run with 20 μL of the standard solution under the above operating conditions, methacrylic acid and ethyl acrylate are eluted in this order with the resolution between these peaks being not less than 5.

System repeatability: When the test is repeated 6 times with 20 μL of the standard solution under the above operating conditions, the relative standard deviations of the peak areas of methacrylic acid and ethyl acrylate are not more than 2.0%, respectively.

Residue on evaporation   Weigh accurately about 1 g of Methacrylic Acid Copolymer LD, evaporate on a water bath to dryness, and dry at 105°C for 4 hours: the amount of the residue is between 27.0% and 33.0%.

Residue on ignition   Not more than 0.10% (2 g).

Assay   Weigh accurately about 1 g of Methacrylic Acid Copolymer LD, dissolve in 20 mL of ethanol (95) by warming, cool, and titrate with 0.1 mol/L sodium hydroxide VS (indicator: 3 drops of phenolphthalein TS). Perform a blank determination in the same manner, and make any necessary correction.

Each mL of 0.1 mol/L sodium hydroxide VS = 8.609 mg of $C_4H_6O_2$

Containers and storage   Containers—Tight containers.

Administration route   Oral administration.

[Note: This item has been revised in the Japanese edition, but the revision does not require any change to the English text stated in the English edition.]

Change the following as follows:

523388

2,2',2"-Nitrilotriethanol

Triethanolamine

2,2',2"－ニトリロトリエタノール

$C_6H_{15}NO_3$: 149.19

2,2',2"-Nitrilotriethanol consists chiefly of 2,2',2'-nitrilotriethanol, and usually contains diethanolamine and monoethanolamine.

It contains not less than 99.0% and not more than 105.0% expressed as 2,2',2"-nitrilotriethanol ($C_6H_{15}NO_3$), calculated on the anhydrous basis.

Description   2,2',2"-Nitrilotriethanol is a colorless to light yellow, viscous liquid. It has a faint, ammonia-like odor.

It is miscible with water and with ethanol (95).

Identification

(1)   To 1 mL of 2,2',2"-Nitrilotriethanol add 0.1 mL of copper (II) sulfate TS: a blue color develops. To this solution add 5 mL of sodium hydroxide TS, and concentrate to 2 mL by heating: the color of the solution does not change.

(2)   Shake 5 mL of a solution of 2,2',2"-Nitrilotriethanol (1 in 10) with 1 mL of ammonium thiocyanate-cobalt (II) nitrate TS, 5 mL of water and 5 mL of a saturated solution of sodium chloride: a red color develops. Shake the solution with 10 mL of isoamyl alcohol: almost no color develops in the isoamyl alcohol layer.

(3)   Heat gently with 1 mL of 2,2',2"-Nitrilotriethanol: the gas evolved changes moistened red litmus paper to blue.

(4)   Determine the infrared absorption spectrum of 2,2',2"-Nitrilotriethanol as directed in the liquid film method under Infrared Spectrophotometry: it exhibits absorption at the wave numbers of about 3370 cm⁻¹, 2950 cm⁻¹, 1455 cm⁻¹, 1360 cm⁻¹, 1283 cm⁻¹, 1154 cm⁻¹, 1038

cm^{-1} and 884 cm^{-1}.

Refractive index n_D^{20}: 1.481−1.486

Specific gravity d_{25}^{25}: 1.120−1.128

pH   Mix 1.0 g of 2,2',2''-Nitrilotriethanol with 10 mL of water: the pH of this solution is between 10.5 and 11.5.

Purity

   (1)   Clarity of solution−Mix 5 mL of 2,2',2''-Nitrilotriethanol with 15 mL of water: the solution is clear.

   (2)   Heavy metals−Proceed with 1.0 g of 2,2',2''-Nitrilotriethanol according to Method 1, and perform the test. Prepare the control solution with 2.0 mL of Standard Lead Solution (not more than 20 ppm).

   (3)   Iron−Dissolve 2.0 g of 2,2',2''-Nitrilotriethanol in 10 mL of water and 3 mL of hydrochloric acid, add 0.03 g of ammonium peroxodisulfate and 10 mL of 1-butanolic potassium thiocyanate TS, and shake vigorously for 30 seconds: the solution has no more color than the following control solution.

     Control solution: Proceed in the same manner using 1.0 mL of Standard Iron Solution (not more than 5 ppm).

   (4)   Arsenic−Prepare the test solution with 1.0 g of 2,2',2''-Nitrilotriethanol according to Method 1, and perform the test (not more than 2 ppm).

Water   Not more than 0.5% (2 g, direct titration, however instead of methanol for water determination, use 30 mL of methanol for water determination plus 5 g of salicylic acid dissolved).

Residue on ignition   Not more than 0.05% (2 g).

Assay   Weigh accurately about 2 g of 2,2',2''-Nitrilotriethanol, add 75 mL of water, shake, and titrate with 1 mol/L hydrochloric acid VS (indicator: 2 drops of methyl red TS).

       Each mL of 1 mol/L hydrochloric acid VS = 149.2 mg of $C_6H_{15}NO_3$

Containers and storage   Containers−Tight containers.

   Storage−Light resistant.

Administration route   Intravenous injection, general external preparation, sublingual application, insecticide.

Change the following as follows:

105114

Peru Balsam

ペルーバルサム

Peru Balsam is the balsam obtained from the skin part of *Myroxylon pereirae* Klotzsch (*Leguminosae*).

Description   Peru Balsam is a dark brown liquid. It has an odor like vanilla.

It is freely soluble in ethanol (95), partially dissolves in diethyl ether and in petroleum benzine, and practically insoluble in water.

It is clear when the layer is thin, and it does not solidify on standing in air.

Identification   To 0.2 mL of Peru Balsam add 1 mL of chloroform, shake well, spread thinly 1 to 2 drops on the optical plate, and evaporate chloroform in hot wind to obtain a film. Determine the infrared absorption spectrum as directed in the film method under Infrared Spectrophotometry: it exhibits absorption at the wave numbers of about 1717 cm^{-1}, 1636 cm^{-1}, 1450 cm^{-1}, 1271 cm^{-1}, 1026 cm^{-1} and 712 cm^{-1}.

Specific gravity d_{20}^{20}: 1.150－1.170

Acid value   42－76. Weigh accurately about 1 g of Peru Balsam, and determine the end point by potentiometric titration.

Saponification value   230－250. Weigh accurately about 3 g of Peru Balsam, add 30 mL of sodium hydroxide TS and 60 mL of diethyl ether, shake for 2 to 3 minutes, and allow to stand. Filter rapidly the diethyl ether layer after the solution has been separated completely, evaporate the diethyl ether on a water bath, and dry the residue at 100°C for 30 minutes: the mass of the residue (cinnamain) is 42% to 60% of the sampling amount. Dissolve the residue in 25 mL of ethanol (95), transfer to a 200-mL volumetric flask, add exactly 25 mL of 0.5 mol/L potassium hydroxide-ethanol VS, connect a small reflux condenser or an air condenser 6 mm in diameter and 750 mm in length, to the flask, and boil gently for 1 hour with occasional shaking in a water bath. After cooling, add 1 mL of phenolphthalein TS, and immediately titrate the excess sodium hydroxide with 0.5 mol/L hydrochloric acid VS. If the solution is turbid at lower temperature, titration should be done while warm. Separately, perform a blank determination in the same manner, using 25 mL of ethanol (95) as the blank solution. Calculate the saponification value by the following equation:

$$\text{Saponification value} = (a - b) \times 28.05/M$$

M: Mass (g) of the residue (cinnamain)

a: Consumed volume (mL) of 0.5 mol/L hydrochloric acid VS in the blank determination

b: Consumed volume (mL) of 0.5 mol/L hydrochloric acid VS using the residue

Purity

(1)　Foreign matter—Place 5 drops of Peru Balsam in a test tube, and shake with 6 mL of petroleum benzine: the powdered residue, other than the pasty insoluble matter put on the surface of the tube, is not revealed.

(2)　Fatty oil—1.0 g of Peru Balsam dissolves clearly in the solution, in which 3 g of chloral hydrate is dissolved in 2 mL of water.

(3)　Rosin—To 4 mL of the filtrate obtained in (4) add 10 mL of a solution of copper (II) acetate monohydrate (1 in 200), and shake: no green to blue-purple color develops in the petroleum benzine layer.

(4)　Turpentine oil and other balsam—To 2.0 g of Peru Balsam add 10 mL of petroleum benzine, shake vigorously, filter, and evaporate 4 mL of the filtrate below 60°C: the odor of benzaldehyde or turpentine oil is not perceptible in the residue. Dissolve 3 drops of the residue in 10 drops of acetic anhydride, and add 2 drops of sulfuric acid: no purple-red to purple-blue color develops.

Containers and storage　Containers—Tight containers.

Storage—Light-resistant.

Administration route　Rectum vagina urethra application, general external preparation.

Change the following as follows:

105340

Polyoxyethylene Castor Oil

ポリオキシエチレンヒマシ油

Polyoxyethylene Castor Oil is obtained by addition polymerization of castor oil with ethylene oxide. The average added molar number of the ethylene oxide is 3, 10, 20, 35, 40, 50 and 60.

Description Polyoxyethylene Castor Oil occurs as a practically colorless to yellow oily liquid, or a petrolatum-like or waxy substance. It has a faint, characteristic odor.

It is freely soluble in ethanol (95), from soluble to practically insoluble in water, and from slightly soluble to practically insoluble in diethyl ether.

Identification

(1) Shake well with 0.5 g of Polyoxyethylene Castor Oil with 10 mL of water and 5 mL of ammonium thiocyanate-cobalt (II) nitrate TS, then add 5 mL of chloroform, and allow to stand after shaking: a blue color develops in the chloroform layer.

(2) Shake 0.5 g of Polyoxyethylene Castor Oil with 10 mL of water, and add 5 drops of bromine TS: the color of the test solution disappears.

pH Dissolve 1.0 g of Polyoxyethylene Castor Oil in 10 mL of water by warming: the pH of this solution is between 6.0 and 8.0 (for intravenous injection).

Dissolve 1.0 g of Polyoxyethylene Castor Oil in 20 mL of water by warming: the pH of this solution is between 4.5 and 7.5 (for general external preparation).

Acid value Not more than 3.0.

Purity

(1) Clarity and color of solution－Dissolve 1.0 g of Polyoxyethylene Castor Oil in 10 mL of water by warming: the solution is clear and colorless to light yellow in color (limited for intravenous injection).

(2) Heavy metals－Proceed with 1.0 g of Polyoxyethylene Castor Oil according to Method 2, and perform the test. Prepare the control solution with 2.0 mL of Standard Lead Solution (not more than 20 ppm).

(3) Arsenic—Prepare the test solution with 1.0 g of Polyoxyethylene Castor Oil according to Method 3, and perform the test (not more than 2 ppm).

Water Not more than 1.0% (1 g, direct titration).

Residue on ignition Not more than 0.20% (1 g).

Containers and storage Containers—Tight containers.

Administration route Intravenous injection (the average added molar number of the ethylene oxide is about 35), general external preparation.

Change the following as follows:

120053

Polyoxyethylene Glyceryl Monococoate (7 E.O.)

ポリオキシエチレンヤシ油脂肪酸グリセリル (7 E.O.)

Polyoxyethylene Glyceryl Monococoate (7 E.O.) is obtained chiefly by addition polymerization of ethylene oxide with glyceryl monofatty acid originated from coconut oil or palm karnel oil. The average added molar number of the ethylene oxide is about 7.

Description　Polyoxyethylene Glyceryl Monococoate (7 E.O.) is a clear, pale yellow and viscous liquid.

It deposits a solid below 5°C, but it has a fluidity.

Identification

(1)　To 5 mL of a solution of Polyoxyethylene Glyceryl Monococoate (7 E.O.) (1 in 20) add 5 mL of sodium hydroxide TS, boil for 5 minutes, cool, and render the solution acidic with dilute hydrochloric acid: a white turbidity is produced.

(2)　To 10 mL of a solution of Polyoxyethylene Glyceryl Monococoate (7 E.O.) (1 in 20) add 5 mL of ammonium thiocyanate-cobalt (II) nitrate TS, shake well, then shake with 5 mL of chloroform, and allow to stand still: a blue color develops in the chloroform layer.

(3)　Shake 0.5 g of Polyoxyethylene Glyceryl Monococoate (7 E.O.) with 10 mL of water, and add 5 drops of bromine TS: the color of the test solution does not disappear.

Acid value　Not more than 5.

Saponification value　84−100

Hydroxyl value　170−190

Iodine value　Not more than 5.

Purity　Heavy metals−Proceed with 1.0 g of Polyoxyethylene Glyceryl Monococoate (7 E.O.) according to Method 2, and perform the test. Prepare the control solution with 2.0 mL of Standard Lead Solution (not more than 20 ppm).

Loss on drying　Not more than 3.0% (1 g, 105°C, 1 hour).

Residue on ignition　Not more than 1.0% (1 g).

Containers and storage   Containers—Tight containers.
Administration route   General external preparation.

Change the following as follows:

502095

Polyoxyethylene Glyceryl Triisostearate

PEG-5 Glyceryl Triisostearate

トリイソステアリン酸ポリオキシエチレングリセリル

Polyoxyethylene Glyceryl Triisostearate consists mainly of triesters of isostearic acid and polyoxyethylene glycerin.

Description   Polyoxyethylene Glyceryl Triisostearate is a light yellow, oily to light yellow-white, waxy substance. It has a faint, characteristic odor, and a slightly bitter taste.

It is freely soluble in ethanol (95), and slightly soluble in water.

Identification

(1)   To 0.5 g of Polyoxyethylene Glyceryl Triisostearate add 10 mL of water and 5 mL of ammonium thiocyanate-cobalt (II) nitrate TS, shake well, then add 5 mL of chloroform, shake, and allow to stand: a blue color develops in the chloroform layer.

(2)   To 0.5 g of Polyoxyethylene Glyceryl Triisostearate add 10 mL of water and 10 mL of potassium hydroxide TS, boil for 5 minutes, and acidify with dilute hydrochloric acid: a pale yellow, oily liquid separates.

(3)   To 0.5 g of Polyoxyethylene Glyceryl Triisostearate add 10 mL of water, shake, and add 5 drops of bromine TS: the color of the test solution does not disappear.

Acid value   Not more than 15.

Purity

(1)   Heavy metals─Proceed with 1.0 g of Polyoxyethylene Glyceryl Triisostearate according to Method 2, and perform the test. Prepare the control solution with 2.0 mL of Standard Lead Solution (not more than 20 ppm).

(2)   Arsenic─Prepare the test solution with 1.0 g of Polyoxyethylene Glyceryl Triisostearate according to Method 3, and perform the test (not more than 2 ppm).

Loss on drying   Not more than 3.0% (1 g, 105°C, 1 hour).

Residue on ignition   Not more than 1.0% (3 g).

Containers and storage   Containers─Tight containers.

Administration route   General external preparation.

Change the following as follows:

108489

Polyoxyethylene Hydrogenated Castor Oil 5

Polyoxyethylene Glycerin Trioxystearic Acid 5

ポリオキシエチレン硬化ヒマシ油 5

Polyoxyethylene Hydrogenated Castor Oil 5 is a non-ionic surfactant obtained by addition polymerization of hydrogenated oil, obtained by adding hydrogen to castor oil, with ethylene oxide. The average added molar number of the ethylene oxide is about 5.

Description   Polyoxyethylene Hydrogenated Castor Oil 5 is a colorless to pale yellow liquid. It has a faint, characteristic odor.

It is miscible with ethanol (95) and with chloroform, and practically insoluble in water and in diethyl ether.

Identification

(1)   To 0.5 g of Polyoxyethylene Hydrogenated Castor Oil 5 add 10 mL of water and 5 mL of ammonium thiocyanate-cobalt (II) nitrate TS, shake well, then shake with 5 mL of chloroform, and allow to stand: a blue color develops in the chloroform layer.

(2)   To 0.5 g of Polyoxyethylene Hydrogenated Castor Oil 5 add 10 mL of water, shake, and add 5 drops of bromine TS: the color of the test solution does not disappear.

Acid value   Not more than 3.0.

Saponification value   140 – 150

Hydroxyl value   123 – 133

Purity   Heavy metals – Proceed with 1.0 g of Polyoxyethylene Hydrogenated Castor Oil 5 according to Method 2, and perform the test. Prepare the control solution with 2.0 mL of Standard Lead Solution (not more than 20 ppm).

Water   Not more than 3.0% (1 g, direct titration).

Residue on ignition   Not more than 0.10% (1 g).

Containers and storage   Containers – Tight containers.

Administration route   General external preparation.

Change the following as follows:

109891

Polyoxyethylene Hydrogenated Castor Oil 10

Polyoxyethylene Glycerin Trioxystearic Acid 10

ポリオキシエチレン硬化ヒマシ油 10

Polyoxyethylene Hydrogenated Castor Oil 10 is a non-ion surfactant obtained by addition polymerization of hydrogenated oil, obtained by adding hydrogen to castor oil, with ethylene oxide. The average added molar number of the ethylene oxide is about 10.

Description　Polyoxyethylene Hydrogenated Castor Oil 10 is a colorless to pale yellow liquid. It has a faint, characteristic odor and a slightly bitter taste.

It is miscible with ethanol (95), with ethyl acetate and with chloroform.

It is practically insoluble in water and in diethyl ether.

Identification

(1)　To 0.5 g of Polyoxyethylene Hydrogenated Castor Oil 10 add 10 mL of water and 5 mL of ammonium thiocyanate-cobalt (II) nitrate TS, shake well, then shake with 5 mL of chloroform, and allow to stand: a blue color develops in the chloroform layer.

(2)　To 0.5 g of Polyoxyethylene Hydrogenated Castor Oil 10 add 10 mL of water, shake, and add 5 drops of bromine TS: the color of the test solution does not disappear.

Acid value　Not more than 1.0.

Saponification value　$113-127$

Hydroxyl value　$98-118$

Purity

(1)　Heavy metals—Proceed with 1.0 g of Polyoxyethylene Hydrogenated Castor Oil 10 according to Method 2, and perform the test. Prepare the control solution with 2.0 mL of Standard Lead Solution (not more than 20 ppm).

(2)　Arsenic—Prepare the test solution with 1.0 g of Polyoxyethylene Hydrogenated Castor Oil 10 according to Method 3, and perform the test (not more than 2 ppm).

Water　Not more than 2.0% (1 g, direct titration).

Residue on ignition　Not more than 0.10% (1 g).

Containers and storage   Containers—Tight containers.
Administration route   General external preparation.

Change the following as follows:

110371

Polyoxyethylene Hydrogenated Castor Oil 20

Polyoxyethylene Glycerin Trioxystearic Acid 20

ポリオキシエチレン硬化ヒマシ油 20

Polyoxyethylene Hydrogenated Castor Oil 20 is a non-ion surfactant obtained by addition polymerization of hydrogenated oil, obtained by adding hydrogen to castor oil, with ethylene oxide. The average added molar number of the ethylene oxide is about 20.

Description   Polyoxyethylene Hydrogenated Castor Oil 20 is a colorless to pale yellow, viscous liquid or a white to pale yellow, petrolatum-like substance. It has a faint, characteristic odor.

It is miscible with ethanol (95) and with ethyl acetate.

It is practically insoluble in water and in diethyl ether.

Identification

(1)   To 0.5 g of Polyoxyethylene Hydrogenated Castor Oil 20 add 10 mL of water and 5 mL of ammonium thiocyanate-cobalt (II) nitrate TS, shake well, then shake with 5 mL of 1-butanol, and allow to stand: a blue color develops in the 1-butanol layer.

(2)   To 0.5 g of Polyoxyethylene Hydrogenated Castor Oil 20 add 10 mL of water, shake, and add 5 drops of bromine TS: the color of the test solution does not disappear.

pH   Shake 1.0 g of Polyoxyethylene Hydrogenated Castor Oil 20 with 20 mL of water by warming: the pH of this solution is between 4.5 and 8.0.

Acid value   Not more than 1.0.

Saponification value   87－97

Hydroxyl value   76－90

Purity   Heavy metals－Proceed with 1.0 g of Polyoxyethylene Hydrogenated Castor Oil 20 according to Method 2, and perform the test. Prepare the control solution with 2.0 mL of Standard Lead Solution (not more than 20 ppm).

Water   Not more than 2.0% (1 g, direct titration).

Residue on ignition   Not more than 0.10% (1 g).

Containers and storage   Containers－Tight containers.

Administration route   General external preparation.

Change the following as follows:

105361

Polyoxyethylene Hydrogenated Castor Oil 40

Polyoxyethylene Glycerin Trioxystearic Acid 40

ポリオキシエチレン硬化ヒマシ油 40

Polyoxyethylene Hydrogenated Castor Oil 40 is a non-ion surfactant obtained by addition polymerization of hydrogenated oil, obtained by adding hydrogen to castor oil, with ethylene oxide. The average added molar number of the ethylene oxide is about 40.

Description   Polyoxyethylene Hydrogenated Castor Oil 40 is a colorless to pale yellow, viscous liquid or a white to pale yellow, petrolatum-like substance. It has a faint, characteristic odor and a slightly bitter taste.

It is very soluble in ethyl acetate and in chloroform, freely soluble in ethanol (95), slightly soluble in water, and practically insoluble in diethyl ether.

Identification

(1)   To 0.5 g of Polyoxyethylene Hydrogenated Castor Oil 40 add 10 mL of water and 5 mL of ammonium thiocyanate-cobalt (II) nitrate TS, shake well, then shake with 5 mL of chloroform, and allow to stand: a blue color develops in the chloroform layer.

(2)   To 0.5 g of Polyoxyethylene Hydrogenated Castor Oil 40 add 10 mL of water, shake, and add 5 drops of bromine TS: the color of the test solution does not disappear.

Congealing point $19-23°C$

pH   To 1.0 g of Polyoxyethylene Hydrogenated Castor Oil 40 add 20 mL of water, and dissolve by warming: the pH of this solution is between 4.5 and 8.0.

Acid value   Not more than 1.0.

Saponification value $54-66$

Hydroxyl value $50-62$

Purity

(1)   Heavy metals — Proceed with 1.0 g of Polyoxyethylene Hydrogenated Castor Oil 40 according to Method 2, and perform the test. Prepare the control solution with 2.0 mL of Standard Lead Solution (not more than 20 ppm).

(2) Arsenic－Prepare the test solution with 1.0 g of Polyoxyethylene Hydrogenated Castor Oil 40 according to Method 3, and perform the test (not more than 2 ppm).

Water   Not more than 2.0% (1 g, direct titration).

Residue on ignition   Not more than 0.10% (1 g).

Containers and storage   Containers－Tight containers.

Administration route   Oral administration, general external preparation, dental external use and troche use.

Change the following as follows:

105362

Polyoxyethylene Hydrogenated Castor Oil 50

Polyoxyethylene Glycerin Trioxystearic Acid 50

ポリオキシエチレン硬化ヒマシ油 50

Polyoxyethylene Hydrogenated Castor Oil 50 is a non-ion surfactant obtained by addition polymerization of hydrogenated oil, obtained by adding hydrogen to castor oil, with ethylene oxide. The average added molar number of the ethylene oxide is about 50.

Description   Polyoxyethylene Hydrogenated Castor Oil 50 is a white to pale yellow, petrolatum-like substance. It has a faint, characteristic odor and a slightly bitter taste.

It is very soluble in ethyl acetate and in chloroform, freely soluble in ethanol (95), slightly soluble in water, and practically insoluble in diethyl ether.

Identification

(1)   To 0.5 g of Polyoxyethylene Hydrogenated Castor Oil 50 add 10 mL of water and 5 mL of ammonium thiocyanate-cobalt (II) nitrate TS, shake well, then shake with 5 mL of chloroform, and allow to stand: a blue color develops in the chloroform layer.

(2)   To 0.5 g of Polyoxyethylene Hydrogenated Castor Oil 50 add 10 mL of water, shake, and add 5 drops of bromine TS: the color of the test solution does not disappear.

Congealing point $23-29°C$

pH   To 1.0 g of Polyoxyethylene Hydrogenated Castor Oil 50 add 20 mL of water, and dissolve by warming: the pH of this solution is between 4.5 and 8.0.

Acid value   Not more than 1.0.

Saponification value $48-58$

Hydroxyl value $42-55$

Purity

(1)   Heavy metals—Proceed with 1.0 g of Polyoxyethylene Hydrogenated Castor Oil 50 according to Method 2, and perform the test. Prepare the control solution with 2.0 mL of Standard Lead Solution (not more than 20 ppm).

(2)   Arsenic—Prepare the test solution with 1.0 g of Polyoxyethylene Hydrogenated Castor

Oil 50 according to Method 3, and perform the test (not more than 2 ppm).

Water　Not more than 3.0% (1 g, direct titration).

Residue on ignition　Not more than 0.10% (1 g).

Containers and storage　Containers—Tight containers.

Administration route　Intravenous injection, intramuscular injection, general external preparation, subcutaneous injection.

Change the following as follows:

108405

Polyoxyethylene Hydrogenated Castor Oil 60

Polyoxyethylene Glycerin Trioxystearic Acid 60

ポリオキシエチレン硬化ヒマシ油 60

Polyoxyethylene Hydrogenated Castor Oil 60 is a non-ion surfactant obtained by addition polymerization of hydrogenated oil, obtained by adding hydrogen to castor oil, with ethylene oxide. The average added molar number of the ethylene oxide is about 60.

Description   Polyoxyethylene Hydrogenated Castor Oil 60 is a white to pale yellow, petrolatum-like or waxy substance. It has a faint, characteristic odor and a slightly bitter taste.

It is very soluble in ethyl acetate and in chloroform, freely soluble in ethanol (95), slightly soluble in water, and practically insoluble in diethyl ether.

Identification

(1)   To 0.5 g of Polyoxyethylene Hydrogenated Castor Oil 60 add 10 mL of water and 5 mL of ammonium thiocyanate-cobalt (II) nitrate TS, shake well, then shake with 5 mL of chloroform, and allow to stand: a blue color develops in the chloroform layer.

(2)   To 0.5 g of Polyoxyethylene Hydrogenated Castor Oil 60 add 10 mL of water, shake, and add 5 drops of bromine TS: the color of the test solution does not disappear.

Congealing point   30－34°C

pH   To 1.0 g of Polyoxyethylene Hydrogenated Castor Oil 60 add 20 mL of water, and dissolve by warming: the pH of this solution is between 4.1 and 7.0.

Acid value   Not more than 1.0.

Saponification value   41－51

Hydroxyl value   39－49

Purity

(1)   Heavy metals－Proceed with 1.0 g of Polyoxyethylene Hydrogenated Castor Oil 60 according to Method 2, and perform the test. Prepare the control solution with 2.0 mL of Standard Lead Solution (not more than 20 ppm).

(2)   Arsenic－Prepare the test solution with 1.0 g of Polyoxyethylene Hydrogenated Castor

Oil 60 according to Method 3, and perform the test (not more than 2 ppm).

Water　Not more than 2.0% (1 g, direct titration).

Residue on ignition　Not more than 0.10% (1 g).

Containers and storage　Containers—Tight containers.

Administration route　Oral administration, intravenous injection, intramuscular injection, subcutaneous injection, intraspinal injection, general external preparation, percutaneous, sublingual application, rectum vagina urethra application, ophthalmic preparation, dental external use and troche use.

Change the following as follows:

120351

Polyoxyethylene Hydrogenated Castor Oil 100

Polyoxyethylene Glycerin Trioxystearic Acid 100

ポリオキシエチレン硬化ヒマシ油 100

Polyoxyethylene Hydrogenated Castor Oil 100 is a non-ion surfactant obtained by addition polymerization of hydrogenated oil, obtained by adding hydrogen to castor oil, with ethylene oxide. The average added molar number of the ethylene oxide is about 100.

Description   Polyoxyethylene Hydrogenated Castor Oil 100 is a white to pale yellow, petrolatum-like or waxy substance. It has a faint, characteristic odor.

It is very soluble in ethyl acetate, freely soluble in water and in ethanol (95), and practically insoluble in diethyl ether.

Identification

(1)   To 0.5 g of Polyoxyethylene Hydrogenated Castor Oil 100 add 10 mL of water and 5 mL of ammonium thiocyanate-cobalt (II) nitrate TS, shake well, then shake with 5 mL of 1-butanol, and allow to stand: a blue color develops in the 1-butanol layer.

(2)   To 0.5 g of Polyoxyethylene Hydrogenated Castor Oil 100 add 10 mL of water, shake, and add 5 drops of bromine TS: the color of the test solution does not disappear.

Congealing point   38−44°C

pH   Dissolve 1.0 g of Polyoxyethylene Hydrogenated Castor Oil 100 in 20 mL of water by warming: the pH of this solution is between 4.5 and 8.0.

Acid value   Not more than 1.0.

Saponification value   29−35

Hydroxyl value   28−38

Purity   Heavy metals−Proceed with 1.0 g of Polyoxyethylene Hydrogenated Castor Oil 100 according to Method 2, and perform the test. Prepare the control solution with 2.0 mL of Standard Lead Solution (not more than 20 ppm).

Water   Not more than 2.0% (1 g, direct titration).

Residue on ignition   Not more than 0.10% (1 g).

Containers and storage Containers—Tight containers.
Administration route Other external use.

Change the following as follows:

105345

Polyoxyl 35 Castor Oil

ポリオキシル 35 ヒマシ油

Polyoxyl 35 Castor Oil is a non-ionic surfactant obtained by addition polymerization of castor oil with ethylene oxide. The average added molar number of the ethylene oxide is about 35.

Description　Polyoxyl 35 Castor Oil occurs as pale yellow to yellow viscous liquid or petrolatum-like or waxy substance. It has a slightly characteristic odor.

　　It is soluble in water, and miscible with ethanol (95).

Identification

　(1)　Melt Polyoxyl 35 Castor Oil by warming if necessary, perform the test as directed in the liquid film method under Infrared Spectrophotometry, and compare the spectrum with the Reference Spectrum: both spectra exhibit similar intensities of absorption at the same wave numbers.

　(2)　Dissolve 0.1 g of Polyoxyl 35 Castor Oil in 10 mL of dilute potassium hydroxide-ethanol TS, and evaporate on a water bath to dryness. Dissolve the residue in 5 mL of water, and add acetic acid (100) dropwise: a white precipitate is formed.

　(3)　To 0.5 g of Polyoxyl 35 Castor Oil add 10 mL of water, dissolve by warming, cool, and add 5 drops of bromine TS: the color of the test solution disappears.

Viscosity　650－850 mPa·s (Method 1, 25°C).

Specific gravity　d^{25}_{25}: 1.05－1.06

Acid value　Not more than 2.0.

Saponification value　60－75

Hydroxyl value　65－80

Iodine value　25－35

Purity

　(1)　Heavy metals－Proceed with 2.0 g of Polyoxyl 35 Castor Oil according to Method 2, and perform the test. Prepare the control solution with 2.0 mL of Standard Lead Solution (not more than 10 ppm).

(2)   Ethylene oxide and 1,4-dioxane－Weigh accurately about 1 g of Polyoxyl 35 Castor Oil, place in a vial, add exactly 1 mL of water, and immediately stopper tightly. Shake the vial to make the contents uniform, warm at 70°C for 45 minutes, and use the contents as the sample solution. Separately, weigh exactly 2 mL of Standard Ethylene Oxide Solution, 0.1 mg/mL, add water to make exactly 100 mL, and use this solution as the standard ethylene oxide stock solution (2 µg/mL). Weigh exactly 1.00 g of 1,4-dioxane, and dissolve in water to make exactly 100 mL. Pipet 5 mL of this solution, and add water to make exactly 50 mL. Pipet 5 mL of this solution, add water to make exactly 50 mL, and use this solution as the standard 1,4-dioxane stock solution (0.1 mg/mL). Weigh accurately about 1 g of Polyoxyl 35 Castor Oil, place in a vial, add exactly 0.5 mL each of the standard ethylene oxide stock solution (2 µg/mL) and standard 1,4-dioxane stock solution (0.1 mg/mL), and immediately stopper tightly. Shake the vial to make the contents uniform, warm at 70°C for 45 minutes, and use the contents as the standard solution. Perform the test with exactly 1 mL each of the vapor phase of the sample solution and standard solution in the vials as directed under Gas Chromatography according to the following conditions, and determine the peak area, A_{T1} and A_{S1}, of ethylene oxide and the peak area, A_{T2} and A_{S2}, of 1,4-dioxane. Calculate the amounts of ethylene oxide and 1,4-dioxane by the following equation: not more than 1 ppm and not more than 10 ppm, respectively.

$$\text{Amount (ppm) of ethylene oxide} = \frac{A_{T1} \times C_1}{A_{S1} \times M_T - A_{T1} \times M_S}$$

$$\text{Amount (ppm) of 1,4-dioxane} = \frac{A_{T2} \times C_2}{A_{S2} \times M_T - A_{T2} \times M_S}$$

M_T: Amount (g) of the sample used in the sample solution

M_S: Amount (g) of the sample used in the standard solution

C_1: Amount (µg) of ethylene oxide added to the standard solution

C_2: Amount (µg) of 1,4-dioxane added to the standard solution

Operating conditions－

Detector: A hydrogen flame-ionization detector.

Column: A fused silica column 0.32 mm in inside diameter and 30 m in length, coated inside with polymethylsiloxan for gas chromatography in 1.0 µm thickness.

Column temperature: Inject at a constant temperature of around 50°C, keep the temperature for 5 minutes, raise the temperature to 180°C at a rate of 5°C per minute, then raise to 230°C at a rate of 30°C per minute, and maintain at a constant temperature of about 230°C for 5 minutes.

Injection port temperature: 150°C

Detector temperature: 250°C

Carrier gas: Helium.

Flow rate: Adjust so that the retention time of 1,4-dioxane is about 9 minutes.

Split ratio: 1:20

System suitability—

Test for required detectability: Place 1.0 g of Polyoxyl 35 Castor Oil in a vial, add exactly 0.8 mL of water, 0.1 mL of the standard ethylene oxide stock solution (2 μg/mL) and 0.1 mL of the standard 1,4-dioxane stock solution (0.1 mg/mL), and immediately stopper tightly. Shake the vial to make the contents uniform, warm at 70°C for 45 minutes, and use the contents as the solution for system suitability test (1). Confirm that the value of the peak areas of ethylene oxide and 1,4-dioxane obtained from the solution for system suitability test (1) subtracted from those from the sample solutions is equivalent to 15 to 25% of the value of the peak areas from the standard solution subtracted from those from the sample solution, respectively.

System performance: Place 0.5 mL of the standard ethylene oxide stock solution (2 μg/mL) in a vial, add 0.1 mL of a solution of acetaldehyde (1 in 100,000), and immediately stopper tightly. Shake the vial to make the contents uniform, warm at 70°C for 45 minutes, and use the contents as the solution for system suitability test (2). When the procedure is run with 1 mL of the gas in vapor phase of the solution for system suitability test (2) in the vial under the above operating conditions, acetaldehyde and ethylene oxide are eluted in this order with the resolution between these peaks being not less than 2.0.

System repeatability: When the test is repeated 6 times with 1 mL of the vapor phase of the standard solution under the above operating conditions, the relative standard deviation of the peak area of ethylene oxide is not more than 15% and that of the peak area of 1,4-dioxane is not more than 10%, respectively.

Water   Not more than 3.0% (1 g, direct titration).

Residue on ignition   Not more than 0.3% (2 g).

Containers and storage   Containers—Tight containers.

Storage—Light-resistant.

Administration route   Oral administration.

Polyoxyl 35 Castor Oil

Ultraviolet-visible Reference Spectra

Polyoxyl 35 Castor Oil

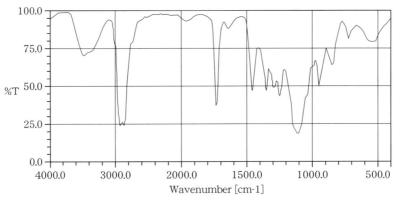

The liquid film method

Change the following as follows:

111794

Polyvinyl Chloride

ポリ塩化ビニル

Polyvinyl Chloride is a straight chain polymer prepared from the suspension polymerization of vinyl chloride ($CH_2=CHCl$), and its mean degree of polymerization is 800 to 1500.

Description   Polyvinyl Chloride occurs as a white powder. It is odorless and tasteless.

It is freely soluble in tetrahydrofuran, and practically insoluble in water, in ethanol (95) and in diethyl ether.

Identification   Determine the infrared absorption spectrum of Polyvinyl Chloride, previously dried, as directed in the potassium bromide disk method under Infrared Spectrophotometry: it exhibits absorption at the wave numbers of about 2950 cm^{-1}, 1420 cm^{-1}, 1240 cm^{-1}, 1070 cm^{-1}, 960 cm^{-1} and 700 cm^{-1}.

Purity   Vinyl chloride－Place 1.0 g of Polyvinyl Chloride in a 20-mL volumetric flask. Add about 10 mL of tetrahydrofuran for gas chromatography, dissolve Polyvinyl Chloride with occasional shaking in a cold place, add tetrahydrofuran for gas chromatography, previously cooled, to make 20 mL while cooling, and use this solution as the sample solution. Perform the test with 2 μL each of the sample solution and the Standard Vinyl Chloride Solution as directed under Gas Chromatography according to the following conditions, and determine the peak heights, H_T and H_S, of vinyl chloride in each solution: H_T is not greater than H_S.

Operating conditions－

Detector: A hydrogen flame-ionization detector.

Column: A column about 3 mm in inside diameter and 2 to 3 m in length, packed with siliceous earth for gas chromatography coated with polypropylene glycol for gas chromatography at the ratio of 10 to 15% (150 to 180 μm in particle diameter).

Column temperature: A constant temperature of 60－70°C.

Carrier gas: Nitrogen.

Flow rate: Adjust so that the retention time of vinyl chloride is about 1.5 minutes.

Selection of column: Proceed with 2 μL of Standard Vinyl Chloride Solution under the above operating conditions. Use a column giving well-resolved peaks of vinyl chloride and ethanol in this order.

Detection sensitivity: Adjust the detection sensitivity so that the peak height of vinyl chloride obtained from 2 μL of Standard Vinyl Chloride Solution is between 50 mm and 70 mm.

Loss on drying　Not more than 1.0% (1 g, 105°C, 2 hours).

Residue on ignition　Not more than 0.5% (1 g).

Containers and storage　Containers－Tight containers.

Administration route　General external preparation.

Change the following as follows:

106968

Sucralose

Trichlorogalactosucrose

スクラロース

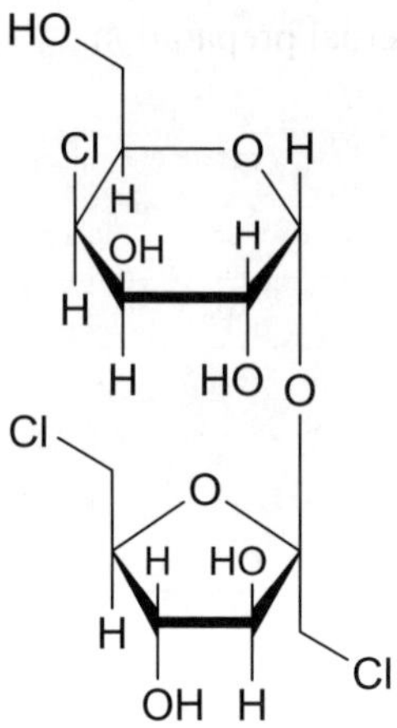

C$_{12}$H$_{19}$Cl$_3$O$_8$: 397.63

Sucralose contains not less than 98.0% and not more than 102.0% of sucralose (C$_{12}$H$_{19}$Cl$_3$O$_8$), calculated on the anhydrous basis.

Description Sucralose occurs as a white to light grayish white, crystalline powder. It is odorless and has a very sweet taste.

It is freely soluble in water and in methanol, and soluble in ethanol (99.5).

Identification

(1) Determine the infrared absorption spectrum of Sucralose as directed in the potassium bromide disk method under Infrared Spectrophotometry, and compare the spectrum with the Reference Spectrum: both spectra exhibit similar intensities of absorption at the same wave numbers.

(2) Dissolve 2.5 g of Sucralose in 10 mL of methanol, and use this solution as the sample solution. Perform the test with this solution as directed under Thin-layer Chromatography. Spot 2 μL of the sample solution on a plate of octadecylsilanized silica gel for thin-layer chromatography. Develop the plate with a mixture of a solution of sodium chloride (1 in 20) and acetonitrile (7:3) to a distance of about 15 cm, and air-dry the plate. Spray evenly diluted sulfuric acid (3 in 20) on the plate, and heat at 125°C for 10 minutes: a black spot is observed at an Rf value of about 0.4 to 0.6.

Optical rotation $[\alpha]_D^{20}$: +84.0−+87.5° (calculated on the anhydrous basis, 1 g, water, 10 mL, 10 mm)

Purity

(1)   Clarity and color of solution−Dissolve 1.0 g of Sucralose in 10 mL of water: the solution is clear and colorless.

(2)   Heavy metals−Proceed with 1.0 g of Sucralose according to Method 2, and perform the test. Prepare the control solution with 1.0 mL of Standard Lead Solution (not more than 10 ppm).

(3)   Related substances−

(i)   Other chlorinated disaccharides: Dissolve 2.5 g of Sucralose in 10 mL of methanol, and use this solution as the sample solution. Pipet 0.5 mL of this solution, add methanol to make exactly 100 mL, and use this solution as the standard solution. Perform the test with these solutions as directed under Thin-layer Chromatography. Spot 2 μL each of the sample solution and standard solution on a plate of octadecylsilanized silica gel for thin-layer chromatography. Develop the plate with a mixture of a solution of sodium chloride (1 in 20) and acetonitrile (7:3) to a distance of about 15 cm, and air-dry the plate. Spray evenly diluted sulfuric acid (3 in 20) on the plate, and heat at 125°C for 10 minutes: the spots other than the principal spot obtained from the sample solution are not more intense than the spot from the standard solution (not more than 0.5%).

(ii)   Chlorinated monosaccharides: Weigh exactly 2.5 g of Sucralose, add exactly 10 mL of methanol to dissolve, and use this solution as the sample solution. Separately, weigh 10.0 g of D-mannitol, dissolve in water to make exactly 100 mL, and use this solution as the standard solution (1). Separately, weigh 10.0 g of D-mannitol and 40.0 mg of fructose, dissolve in water to make exactly 100 mL, and use this solution as the standard solution (2). Spot 5 μL each of the sample solution, and the standard solutions (1) and (2) on a plate of silica gel for thin-layer chromatography. Spray evenly p-anisidine-phthalic acid TS, and heat between 98°C and 102°C for about 10 minutes. After heating, immediately observe against a black background: the spot from the sample solution is not more intense than the spot from the standard solution (2). When a black spot develops in the standard solution (1), shorten the time for heating, and perform the test again (not more than 0.16% as fructose).

(4) Triphenylphosphine oxide－Weigh accurately about 0.1 g of Sucralose, dissolve in the mobile phase to make exactly 10 mL, and use this solution as the sample solution. Separately, weigh accurately about 0.1 g of triphenylphosphine oxide, and dissolve in the mobile phase to make exactly 10 mL. Pipet 1 mL of this solution, and add the mobile phase to make exactly 100 mL. Further, pipet 1 mL of this solution, add the mobile phase to make exactly 100 mL, and use this solution as the standard solution. Perform the test with exactly 25 μL each of the sample solution and standard solution as directed under Liquid Chromatography according to the following conditions. Determine the peak area, A_T and A_S, of triphenylphosphine oxide in each solution, and calculate the amount of triphenylphosphine oxide by the following formula: it is not more than 150 ppm.

$$\text{Amount (ppm) of triphenylphosphine oxide (}C_{18}H_{15}OP) = \frac{M_S}{M_T} \times \frac{A_T}{A_S} \times 100$$

M_S: Amount (g) of triphenylphosphine oxide
M_T: Amount (g) of sample

Operating conditions －

Detector: An ultraviolet absorption photometer (wavelength: 220 nm).

Column: A stainless steel column 4.6 mm in inside diameter and 15 cm in length, packed with octadecylsilanized silica gel for liquid chromatography (5 μm in particle diameter).

Column temperature: A constant temperature of about 40°C.

Mobile phase: A mixture of acetonitrile for liquid chromatography and water (67:33).

Flow rate: Adjust so that the retention time of triphenylphosphine oxide is about 2 minutes.

(5) Methanol－Weigh accurately about 0.25 g of methanol, add water to make exactly 100 mL, and use this solution as the standard stock solution. Separately, weigh accurately about 0.25 g of *t*-butyl alcohol, dissolve in water to make exactly 100 mL, and use this solution as the internal standard stock solution. Pipet 2 mL of the internal standard stock solution, add water to make exactly 250 mL, and use this solution as the internal standard solution. Further pipet 10 mL of the standard stock solution, add exactly 2 mL of the internal standard stock solution, add water to make exactly 250 mL, and use this solution as the standard solution. Pipet 10 mL of the standard solution, and transfer to a headspace vial. Transfer about 1.0 g of Sucralose, accurately weighed, to another headspace vial in the same manner, add exactly 10 mL of the internal standard solution, and use this solution as the test solution.

Perform the test with the standard solution and test solution as directed in the headspace method under Gas Chromatography according to the following conditions, and calculate the ratios, Q_S and Q_T, of the peak area of methanol to that of t-butyl alcohol in each solution. Calculate the amount of methanol by the following equation: it is not more than 0.1%.

$$\text{Amount (\%) of methanol} = \frac{M_S}{M_T} \times \frac{Q_T}{Q_S} \times \frac{2}{5}$$

M_S: Amount (g) of methanol

M_T: Amount (g) of sample

Head-space sampler conditions —

Equilibration temperature in vial: 60°C

Equilibration time in vial: 20 minutes

Transfer line temperature: 180°C

Syringe temperature: 100°C

Pressurization: 115 kPa, Pressurization time: 1 minute, Injection time: 0.05 minute (follow the instrument manufacture's recommendations, as long as the method criteria are met. A difference in injection is allowed as long as adequate sensitivity is achieved.)

Operating conditions —

Detector: A hydrogen flame-ionization detector.

Column: A fused silica tube 0.53 mm in inside diameter and 60 m in length, coated with 6% cyanopropyl phenyl-94% dimethyl silicone polymer for gas chromatography in 3.0 μm thickness.

Column temperature: Maintain at 40°C for 1 minute, raise to 60°C at 5°C per minute, then raise to 240°C at 40°C per minute, and maintain at 240°C for 5 minutes.

Carrier gas: Helium.

Injection port temperature: A constant temperature of about 180°C.

Column temperature: A constant temperature of around 250°C.

Split ratio: Splitless.

Flow rate: Adjust so that the retention time of methanol is about 2 minutes.

System suitability —

System performance: When the procedure is run with the standard solution under above operating conditions, methanol and t-butyl alcohol are eluted in this order with the resolution between these peaks being not less than 5.

System repeatability: When the test is repeated 6 times with the standard solution under the above operating conditions, the relative standard deviation of the ratio of the peak area of methanol to that of *t*-butyl alcohol is not more than 2.0%.

Water   Not more than 2.0% (1 g, volumetric titration, direct titration).

Residue on ignition   Not more than 0.7% (1 g).

Assay   Weigh accurately about 1 g of Sucralose, calculated on the anhydrous basis, and dissolve in water to make exactly 100 mL. Pipet 10 mL of this solution, add 10 mL of a solution of sodium hydroxide (1 in 10), and boil gently under a reflux condenser for 30 minutes. After cooling, neutralize with dilute nitric acid, and titrate with 0.1 mol/L silver nitrate VS (potentiometric titration). Perform a blank determination in the same manner, and make any necessary correction.

Each mL of 0.1 mol/L silver nitrate VS = 13.25 mg of $C_{12}H_{19}Cl_3O_8$

Containers and storage   Containers—Well-closed containers.

Storage—In a cold place (1 to 20°C).

Administration route   Oral administration.

Ultraviolet-visible Reference Spectra

Sucralose

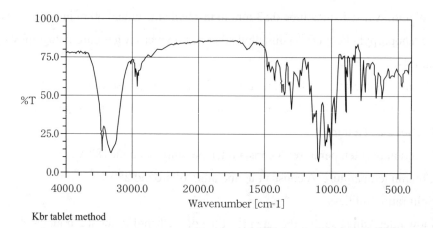

Kbr tablet method

Change the following as follows:

109280

α-Thioglycerol

アルファチオグリセリン

C$_3$H$_8$O$_2$S: 108.16

α-Thioglycerol contains not less than 98.0% of α-Thioglycerol (C$_3$H$_8$O$_2$S), calculated on the anhydrous basis.

Description   α-Thioglycerol is clear, colorless to light yellow and viscous liquid. It has a characteristic odor.

It is miscible with water and with ethanol (95), and practically insoluble in diethyl ether.

Identification   To 5 mL a solution of α-Thioglycerol (1 in 100) add 2 mL of sodium hydroxide TS and 1 mL of lead acetate TS, and heat on a water bath: a black precipitate is formed.

Refractive index n_D^{20}: 1.521$-$1.526

pH   Dissolve 1.0 g of α-Thioglycerol in 10 mL of water: the pH of this solution is between 3.5 and 7.0.

Specific gravity d_{25}^{25}: 1.241$-$1.250

Purity

(1)   Clarity and color of solution$-$Dissolve 1.0g of α-Thioglycerol in 10 mL of water: the solution is clear and colorless.

(2)   Heavy metals$-$Proceed with 1.0g of α-Thioglycerol according to Method 2, and perform the test. Prepare the control solution with 2.0 mL of Standard Lead Solution (not more than 20 ppm).

(3)   Arsenic$-$Prepare the test solution with 1.0 g of α-Thioglycerol according to Method 1, and perform the test (not more than 2 ppm).

Water   Not more than 2.0% (0.5 g, direct titration, however instead of methanol for water determination, use 30 mL of methanol for water determination plus 10 g of *N*-ethylmaleimide dissolved).

Residue on ignition   Not more than 0.10% (1 g).

Assay   Weigh accurately about 0.4 g of α-Thioglycerol, dissolve in 50 mL of water, and titrate with 0.50 mol/L iodine VS (indicator: 3 mL of starch TS).

$$\text{Each mL of 0.05 mol/L iodine VS} = 10.816 \text{ mg of } C_3H_8O_2S$$

Containers and storage   Containers－Tight containers.

Administration route   Intravenous injection, intramuscular injection, subcutaneous injection.

Change the following as follows:

004408

Triacetine

トリアセチン

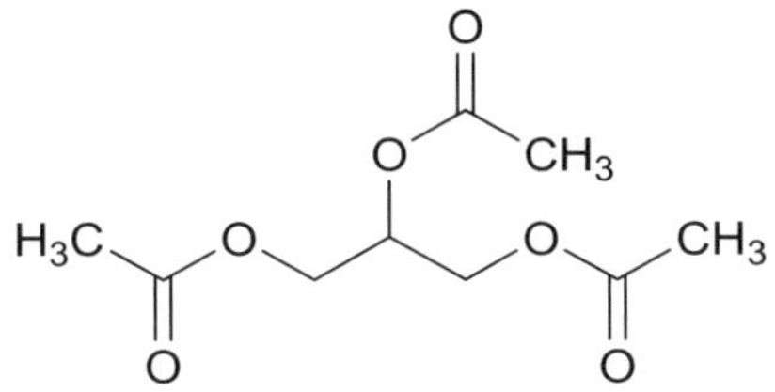

$C_9H_{14}O_6$: 218.20

Triacetine contains not less than 99.0% of triacetine ($C_9H_{14}O_6$).

Description　Triacetine is a colorless, slightly viscous liquid. It is odorless, and has a bitter taste.

　　It is miscible with ethanol (95).

　　It is soluble in water.

　　Boiling point: 257－260°C

Identification　To several drops of Triacetine add a small quantity of ethanol (95) and sulfuric acid, and heat: the odor of ethyl acetate is perceptible.

Refractive index　n_D^{20}: 1.430－1.432

Specific gravity　d_{20}^{20}: 1.158－1.164

Purity

　(1)　Acidity－To 40.0 g of Triacetine add 40 mL of neutralized ethanol, shake, and add 0.20 mL of 0.1 mol/L potassium hydroxide-ethanol VS and 3 drops of phenolphthalein TS: the color of the solution is red.

　(2)　Heavy metals－Dissolve 4.0 g of Triacetine in 10 mL of ethanol (95), proceed according to Method 1, and perform the test. Prepare the control solution with 2.0 mL of Standard Lead solution (not more than 5 ppm).

　(3)　Arsenic－Prepare the test solution with 1.0 g of Triacetine according to Method 1, and perform the test (not more than 2 ppm).

Water　Not more than 0.15% (5 g, direct titration).

Assay   Weigh accurately about 1 g of Triacetine, add exactly 40 mL of 0.5 mol/L potassium hydroxide-ethanol VS, shake frequently under a reflux condenser in a water bath between 60°C and 65°C, and heat gently for 1.5 to 2 hours. After cooling, titrate immediately the excess potassium hydroxide with 0.25 mol/L sulfuric acid VS (indicator: 3 drops of phenolphthalein TS). If turbidity is produced, dissolve it by warming, and titrate. Perform a blank determination in the same manner.

Each mL of 0.5 mol/L potassium hydroxide-ethanol VS = 36.367 mg of $C_9H_{14}O_6$

Containers and storage   Containers — Tight containers.

Administration route   Oral administration, general external preparation, dental external use and troche use.

Change the following as follows:

107647

Wheat Germ Oil

小麦胚芽油

Wheat Germ Oil is the fixed oil obtained from the germ of *Triticum aestivum* Linné (*Gramdneae*).

Description Wheat Germ Oil is a clear, light yellow oil. It has a faint, characteristic odor and a mild taste.

It is miscible with diethyl ether and with cyclohexane.

It is slightly soluble in ethanol (95), and practically insoluble in water.

Identification To 0.5 g of Wheat Germ Oil add 10 mL of potassium hydroxide-ethanol TS, heat gently on a water bath under a reflux condenser for 1 hour with occasional shaking. After cooling, add 7 mL of dilute hydrochloric acid, 40 mL of water and 30 mL of chloroform, and extract by vigorous shaking. Separate the chloroform layer, evaporate the chloroform, dissolve the residue in 0.5 mL of ethanol (95), and use this solution as the sample solution. To 1 drop of the sample solution add 1 drop of a saturated solution of hydroxylammonium chloride in ethanol (95) and 1 drop of *N,N'*-dicyclohexylcarbodiimide-ethanol TS, allow to stand at room temperature for more than 1 minute, and add 1 drop of a mixture of iron (III) chloride-methanol TS and hydrochloric acid (1000:1): a red-purple color develops immediately.

Specific gravity d_{25}^{25}: $0.912-0.932$

Acid value Not more than 1.0.

Saponification value $182-194$

Unsaponifiable matter Not more than 6.0%.

Iodine value $125-140$

Purity

(1) Heavy metals—Proceed with 1.0 g of Wheat Germ Oil according to Method 2, and perform the test. Prepare the control solution with 2.0 mL of Standard Lead Solution (not more than 20 ppm).

(2) Arsenic—To 1.0 g of Wheat Germ Oil in a porcelain crucible add 10 mL of a solution of magnesium nitrate hexahydrate in ethanol (99.5) (1 in 10), fire the ethanol to burn, and heat

gradually to incinerate. After cooling, to the residue add 10 mL of dilute hydrochloric acid, dissolve by warming on a water bath, and perform the test with this solution (not more than 2 ppm).

Residue on ignition   Not more than 0.10% (1 g).

Containers and storage   Containers — Tight containers.

Administration route   Oral administration.

INDEX

INDEX IN JAPANESE